Contemporary Diagnosis
and Management of

Hypertension®

Myron H. Weinberger, MD
Director, Hypertension Research Center
Indiana University School of Medicine
Indianapolis, Indiana

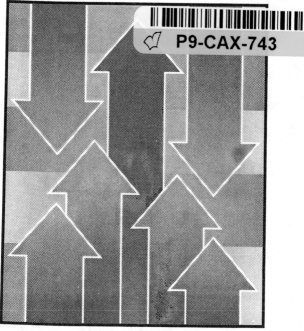

P9-CAX-743

First Edition

Published by Handbooks in Health Care Co., Newtown, Pennsylvania, USA

International Standard Book Number: 1-884065-14-7

Library of Congress Catalog Card Number: 96-79872

Table of Contents

This book has been prepared and is presented as a service to the medical community. The information provided reflects the knowledge, experience, and personal opinions of Myron H. Weinberger, MD, Professor of Medicine, and Director, Hypertension Research Center, Indiana University School of Medicine, Indianapolis.

This book is not intended to replace or to be used as a substitute for the complete prescribing information prepared by each manufacturer for each drug. Because of possible variations in drug indications, in dosage information, in newly described toxicities, in drug/drug interactions, and in other items of importance, reference to such complete prescribing information is definitely recommended before any of the drugs discussed are used or prescribed.

Chapter 1

Definition, Epidemiology, Natural History, and Benefits of Treatment

Hypertension is arbitrarily defined as a *persistent* elevation of blood pressure that exceeds 140 mm Hg systolic and/or 90 mm Hg diastolic when indirectly measured with a sphygmomanometer.[1] The fifth Korotkoff phase (disappearance of sound) has been used for the diastolic pressure. Although these criteria are applied in the United States, the World Health Organization (WHO) established a level of 160/95 mm Hg as that which requires treatment. The 1997 report of the Joint National Committee (JNC) on Detection, Evaluation and Treatment of High Blood Pressure indicates that a diastolic pressure of 85 to 89 mm Hg or a systolic pressure of 130 to 139 mm Hg are considered high normal values, and that patients with such values merit scrutiny because they are more likely to develop fixed hypertension with time.[1] For the greatest accuracy, blood pressure should be measured after the subject is seated for 5 minutes and with the patient's arm at heart level. Because a cold environment can elevate pressure, room temperature should be normal. The blood pressure cuff size should be appropriate for arm circumference, because the use of a cuff too small for arm size can produce an artificial elevation of blood pressure. Most sphygmomanometer cuffs made in the past 20 years have a gauge inside the cuff to indicate if the size is appropriate for an individual's arm. If the blood pressure is markedly elevated (ie, systolic

>210 mm Hg, diastolic >120 mm Hg), immediate evaluation and intervention are indicated. Lower values should be confirmed with a repeat measurement after a week or more before additional evaluation is initiated. When target organ disease (see Chapter 3) is present, a more aggressive approach is indicated.

Epidemiology

The prevalence of hypertension varies considerably, based on geographic, cultural, demographic, nutritional, and genetic factors. It is more common in industrial societies than in primitive cultures, varying in frequency from more than 25% of the adult American population to nonexistent among the Yanomamo Indians of the Amazon jungle. According to results of migration studies, industrialization and acculturation of isolated peoples are associated with a marked increase in the prevalence of hypertension. The cause of this change is not clear. Some experts implicate the relationship to a change in traditional nutritional habits from a diet usually low in sodium and high in potassium and calcium, because hypertension is more common with a relatively high-salt, low-potassium, low-calcium diet typical of industrial societies. Evidence to support this contention can be inferred from several intervention studies. Among the Samburu of Kenya, whose native diet is high in potassium and low in sodium, blood pressure levels are typically low or normal. When young men of this tribe are recruited into the Kenyan army and given a high-sodium, low-potassium diet, their blood pressure increases markedly. The army life-style, of course, differs from their typical environment in other ways as well, but when these men return to their native life-style and diet after leaving the army, blood pressure levels decrease to pre-army values. However, we cannot identify which component(s) may be responsible for the change in blood pressure.

Another cultural observation to support the diet/blood pressure relationship occurred in Japan. Before 1970, the

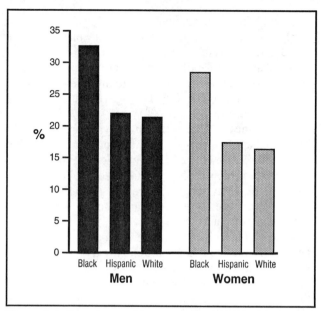

Figure 1-1: Prevalence of hypertension (>140/90) NHANES III (age 18-74) (Data from: *Hypertension* 1995;26:60).

salt intake of the northern Japanese was among the highest in the world, averaging 15 to 20 g per day. This population also had the highest prevalence of hypertension known at that time, observed in approximately 40% of the adults. The leading cause of death was cerebral hemorrhage. A public health campaign was mounted to educate the people both to reduce salt intake by changing some of the methods of preparing and preserving food, and to increase intake of potassium and calcium. Results of subsequent surveys demonstrated a significant decrease in the prevalence of hypertension and stroke. However, these observations do not directly implicate salt as the causative factor. Results of other studies that show a strong interaction between increased salt intake and reduced potassium and calcium intake and both blood pressure and cardiovascular disease imply that the ratios of these nutrients may play a role. But not all individuals in a given population demonstrate blood pressure that is susceptible to these nutritional components. In addition, there is now evidence to indicate that the susceptibility of blood pressure to changes in salt balance may increase with age.

Obesity has also been linked to hypertension, a relationship that often persists after the confounding element of blood pressure cuff size is remedied. The mechanisms responsible for this association are not clear. Other factors such as stress, environmental crowding, physical inactivity, and other life-style factors are associated with blood pressure elevation.

Even within a given population, marked differences can be observed in the risk for developing hypertension. For example, African Americans, with a prevalence as high as 40%, are more likely to have or to develop hypertension than are Native Americans, Hispanic Americans, or Caucasians (Figure 1-1). The prevalence of hypertension increases with age, so that more than 60% of Americans older than 60 years of age have an elevated diastolic and/or systolic pressure.[1] Isolated systolic hypertension (systolic pressure >140 mm Hg, diastolic pressure < 90 mm Hg) is more common in the elderly population (see Chapter 9).

The familial nature of hypertension has long suggested that it may be inherited. A possible role has been identified for genetic factors because hypertension is more common in some families than in others. A genetic basis was recently described for several relatively unusual forms of hypertension: Liddle's syndrome, dexamethasone- or glucocorticoid-remediable aldosteronism (DRA or GRA), the syndrome of apparent mineralocorticoid excess (AME), and the brachydactyly-hypertension syndrome, all of which are examined in Chapter 3. Although such observations suggest a genetic basis, they could also reflect a shared environment and the contribution of some exogenous component. However, a major genetic component for essential hypertension was confirmed through observations that this form of primary hypertension is more common in both members of identical twin pairs than in fraternal twins. Substantial resources have been committed to the search for the essential hypertension gene. Given the multifactorial basis for blood pressure control and the development of hypertension (discussed in Chapter 2), a polygenic etiology is likely. Recent evidence suggests an inverse relationship between birth weight and blood pressure levels in adulthood, which in turn suggests that premature birth may be yet another risk factor for the development of hypertension.[2]

Natural History and Consequences

Results of numerous studies implicate elevated blood pressure as a major cause of death and disability, primarily by contributing to cardiovascular and renal disease. Actuarial data indicate that the risk attributable to blood pressure is based on a continuum rather than on hierarchical levels, making the definition of elevated blood pressure an arbitrary one. A graded reduction in life expectancy can be shown as the level in untreated individuals increases from 100/60 to 180/100 mm Hg. Thus, the choice of a blood pressure level of 140/90 or 160/95 mm Hg as appropriate for intervention is arbitrary. Recent observations indicate that systolic pressure carries as great a risk, and for some events even a greater risk, than does diastolic pressure. Isolated systolic hypertension, encountered more often in older patients (ie, > 60 years) (see Chapter 9), is associated with all of the cardiovascular consequences of systolic-diastolic hypertension.

The events linked to blood pressure elevation include stroke (the result of cerebral hemorrhage or infarction), dementia, angina and myocardial infarction, peripheral vascular disease, left ventricular hypertrophy and congestive heart failure, cardiac arrhythmias and sudden death, dissecting aneurysms, and renal failure.[3] Cerebral hemorrhage, left ventricular hypertrophy, congestive heart failure, and dissecting aneurysm can be directly related to damage to the vasculature and myocardium induced by the increase in pressure. Cerebral ischemia and infarction, myocardial ischemia and infarction, peripheral vascular disease, and renal failure are the result of ischemia secondary to arterial thickening and constriction. These occur in response to increased pressure or to the process of atherosclerosis, which is accelerated by elevated blood pressure even in the presence of normal lipid and lipoprotein levels. In addition, the increased vasoconstrictor response is associated with a reduction in blood flow, a change in blood to a sludgy consistency, and an increased propensity for blood clotting, particularly if increased levels of fibrinogen are present. Moreover, the presence of increased amounts of the small, dense, low-density lipoprotein (LDL) particles in patients with hypertension, particularly in those with insulin resistance, further enhances the atherosclerotic process.

Results of recent population studies demonstrate a greater frequency in the concurrence of dyslipidemia (defined as an elevation of total cholesterol, triglycerides, or LDLs or a decreased level of high-density lipoproteins) and insulin resistance (carbohydrate intolerance) in patients with hypertension than could be predicted from the prevalence of either condition in the overall population. These observations led to speculation that this may represent a syndrome, possibly genetic, which could account for the enhanced impact of hypertension on cardiovascular risk. When blood pressure elevation occurs in concert with other risk factors for cardiovascular disease–such as dyslipidemia, carbohydrate intolerance or diabetes mellitus, cigarette smoking, or left ventricular hypertrophy–the risk of cardiovascular disease dramatically increases.[4] Unfortunately, most patients with elevated blood pressure also manifest other cardiovascular risk factors, making the typical patient with elevated blood pressure a high-risk subject for cardiovascular disease.

These factors must be considered in the evaluation of the patient with hypertension when deciding whether and how aggressively to treat the patient and when choosing the most appropriate treatment for both the blood pressure and the other risk factors. In addition, more aggressive treatment of all identifiable risk factors is indicated in the individual with manifestations of vascular disease (angina, history of myocardial infarction, transient ischemic attack, stroke, or peripheral vascular disease). Recent evidence, for example, indicates that in patients with a history of myocardial infarction who have lipid levels within the normal range, reducing lipid levels with drugs can decrease the likelihood of recurrence of myocardial infarction or death.

One of the most frustrating aspects of hypertension is its asymptomatic nature. Unless discovered during a routine medical encounter or screening exercise, the individual is often unaware of the presence of elevated blood pressure until sufficient vascular damage occurs as manifested by target organ involvement. For this reason, the routine measurement of blood pressure, an inexpensive, relatively painless, and widely available procedure, should be conducted at every medical encounter, or at least annually in all adults. It should be taken more frequently if there is a family history of hypertension or if the individual is known to be at increased risk for the development of hypertension because of demographic characteristics or health problems.[1] If risk factors such as cigarette smoking, dyslipidemia, carbohydrate intolerance, or left ventricular hypertrophy are known, more frequent evaluation of blood pressure, and a more vigorous approach to treatment of even mild elevations, are appropriate. The JNC VI report provides stratification of antihypertensive therapy based on risk factors and target organ disease, as well as on the level of blood pressure elevation.

When blood pressure is elevated, an increased risk for all of the previously described cardiovascular events can be easily demonstrated. The impact of systolic blood pressure is greater than that of diastolic pressure, although both are important. The benefit of blood pressure reduction in decreasing these events is less uniform. Because the risk of cardiovascular events depends on the severity of blood pressure elevation, the duration of hypertension, the patient's age, the presence of other risk factors, perhaps differences in individual susceptibility to specific vascular events, and pressure-independent effects of antihypertensive drugs, it is not surprising that all of the intervention trials have not yielded similar results. One of the first studies to examine the benefit of treating hypertension, the Veterans Administration Cooperative Study, randomly assigned patients with hypertension whose diastolic blood pressure ranged from 115 to 129 mm Hg to treatment with placebo or a stepped-care drug regimen.[5] This study of patients with severe hypertension was one of the first to demonstrate that reducing blood pressure with antihypertensive drugs significantly reduced morbidity and mortality from cardiovascular disease. Results of subsequent studies of less severe hypertensives also showed a reduction in overall mortality, but most convincingly in stroke. This dramatic and significant decrease in stroke can be seen in almost all other large antihypertensive intervention trials featuring a placebo-treated control group and tends to be evident after a relatively short period of blood pressure reduction.[6]

Less consistent evidence demonstrates that blood pressure reduction with antihypertensive agents, such as diuretics and β-adrenergic blocking drugs, decreases the risk of myocardial infarction, the most common cardiovascular event, or the occurrence of sudden death. Several explanations have been offered for this apparent inconsistency between effects of lowering blood pressure in decreasing stroke versus heart attacks. The first is that hypertension is not a direct risk factor for myocardial infarction; however, this appears to be refuted by the evidence of a continuous increase in risk for this event with increasing levels of systolic or diastolic pressure. Another possible explanation is that whereas stroke is a sudden pressure-related event, myocardial infarction results from a more lengthy process of ischemia, atherosclerosis, plaque rupture, and thrombus formation. Thus, a longer period of antihypertensive therapy may be required to demonstrate reversal or prevention of coronary artery disease than is needed to demonstrate decreased risk for stroke. Another possibility is that adverse effects of antihypertensive agents on other risk factors for myocardial infarction could contribute to the failure to observe dramatic or consistent reductions in myocardial infarction during these intervention trials. These effects include alterations in the lipid profile, carbohydrate intolerance,[7] the coagulation cascade, or excessive reduction of diastolic pressure (the J curve phenomenon).[8] Evidence to support these possibilities is derived indirectly from two large recent studies that demonstrate an increased risk of sudden death in patients with hypertension who were treated with diuretics or β-blocking drugs.[9,10] However, it is clear that blood pressure reduction in patients with hypertension is beneficial in reducing cardiovascular morbidity and mortality, and that the benefit is greatest in those with the most marked elevation of pressure. It is less evident whether the level of blood pressure reduction influences outcome or whether the specific type of drug used for lowering blood pressure makes a difference in the occurrence of specific events.

To address these issues, several large multicenter and multinational trials are in progress. One such trial that has been completed is the Hypertension Optimal Treatment (HOT) Study. This study recruited approximately 18,000 hypertensive patients at centers all over the world to determine whether the reduction of diastolic pressure to levels of 80, 85, or 90 mm Hg has a differential effect on morbidity or mortality from specific cardiovascular events. The study also examined the benefit of aspirin treatment in hypertension. The treatment algorithm for the HOT study began with a dihydropyridine calcium channel blocker, felodipine (Plendil®), to which an ACE inhibitor, β-blocker, or diuretic could be added. The HOT study demonstrated a progressive reduction in cardiovascular events with aggressive reduction of diastolic pressure. The greatest benefit was seen in hypertensives with diabetes mellitus, where the risk of cardiovascular events in those assigned to diastolic pressure of 80 was half that of those assigned to 90. Aspirin was also found to reduce cardiac events in these treated hypertensives without increasing stroke. Studies such as the one jointly sponsored by the National Heart, Lung and Blood Institute and pharmaceutical companies (ALLHAT) are in progress to determine whether blood pressure reduction with specific, different classes of antihypertensive agents, with or without lipid-lowering agents, influence cardiovascular events. Still other studies (such as LIIFE) are directed toward the role of left ventricular hypertrophy reduction in the treatment of hypertension as a factor that influences cardiovascular events. Additional multicenter trials in patients with hypertension and multiple risk factors for cardiovascular disease (CONVINCE, PREDICT, and others) examine the benefit of specific antihypertensive drugs in the reduction of cardiovascular events. Despite the massive efforts involved in these trials, it is unlikely that definitive information concerning the benefits or disadvantages of individual antihypertensive agents will be available until the 21st century.

It is clear that the treatment of elevated blood pressure reduces the risk of developing malignant hypertension or congestive heart failure. However, the benefit of antihypertensive treatment in the prevention of renal failure, at least in the high-risk subgroup represented by African Americans, has not been clearly demonstrated. Studies are in progress to examine this issue (AASK). The incidences of end-stage renal disease and congestive heart failure, both of which are largely caused by elevated blood pressure, have increased dramatically over the past few decades. Certainly, the reduction of elevated blood pressure by a variety of means is associated with a reduction in cardiovascular morbidity and mortality caused by a variety of factors. It also remains to be demonstrated whether specific pharmacologic or nonpharmacologic blood pressure-lowering approaches have different effects on total morbidity or mortality or on specific outcomes of cardiovascular events. A number of trials to examine different aspects of this issue are in progress and may provide more definitive information. The greatest concern now focuses on the 75% of the hypertensive population in whom adequate blood pressure control has not been achieved.[1]

References

1.   Joint National Committee on Prevention, Detection, Evaluation, and Treatment of High Blood Pressure: the sixth report. *Arch Intern Med* 1997;157:2413-2446.

2.   Chertow GM, Brenner BM: Low birth weight as a risk factor for juvenile and adult hypertension. In: Laragh JH, Brenner BM, eds. *Hypertension: Pathophysiology, Diagnosis, and Management,* 2nd ed. New York, Raven Press, 1995, pp 89-97.

3.   Stamler J, Stamler R, Neaton JD: Blood pressure, systolic and diastolic and cardiovascular risks: U.S. population data. *Arch Intern Med* 1993;153:598-615.

4.   Anderson KM, Wilson PW, Odell PM, et al: An updated coronary risk profile. A statement for health professionals. *Circulation* 1991;83:356-362.

5.   Veterans Administration Cooperative Study Group on Antihypertensive Agents: effects of treatment on morbidity in hypertension: results in patients with diastolic pressures averaging 115 through 129 mm Hg. *JAMA* 1967;202:116-122.

6.   Collins R, Peto R, MacMahon S: Blood pressure, stroke, and coronary heart disease. Part 2, Short-term reductions in blood pressure: overview of randomised drug trials in their epidemiological context. *Lancet* 1990;335:827-838.

7.   Weinberger MH: Antihypertensive therapy and lipids: paradoxical influences on cardiovascular disease risk. *Am J Med* 1986;80(2A):64-70.

8.   Cruikshank JM, Thorp JM, Zacharias FJ: Benefits and potential harm of lowering blood pressure. *Lancet* 1987;1:581-584.

9.   Siscovick DS, Ragunathan TE, Psaty BM, et al: Diuretic therapy for hypertension and the risk of primary cardiac arrest. *N Engl J Med* 1994;330:1852-1857.

10. Hoes AW, Grobbee DE, Lubsen J, et al: Diuretics, β-blockers and sudden cardiac death in hypertensive patients. *Ann Intern Med* 1995;123:481-487.

Chapter 2

Pathophysiology of Hypertension

T he human circulatory system is an intricate network of mechanisms designed to maintain homeostasis of pressure and flow despite myriad perturbations.[1] This remarkable system permits physiologic defense, at least temporarily, in the face of dramatic events such as hemorrhage, shock, stress-induced changes, overload of extracellular fluid volume, excessive fluid loss, and other potentially life-threatening events. Thus, a sustained elevation of arterial pressure reflects a disturbance in the delicate balance of factors that maintains this equilibrium. In the case of some secondary forms of hypertension (see Chapter 4), an abnormality in a single component of blood pressure regulation is sometimes sufficient to upset the homeostatic balance and result in hypertension. For most patients with primary (essential) or idiopathic hypertension, subtle abnormalities of more than one factor are involved. Because so many possible factors are involved in primary hypertension and because its evolution is so gradual and subtle, identifying a single causal factor in most patients is usually difficult. Additionally, given the multiplicity of these contributing factors, it is not surprising that the pathophysiology, manifestations, and responses to intervention are so varied among patients.

Evidence of individual differences is readily apparent from the many different antihypertensive agents now

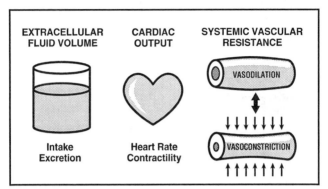

Figure 2-1: Factors that influence blood pressure.

available and from the heterogeneity of blood pressure responses to these agents. Moreover, an understanding of the different factors that contribute to the elevation of blood pressure provides a better basis for recognizing the differences in individual manifestations, complications, and treatment approaches. This chapter reviews these factors by separating the components of blood pressure control into three general mechanisms: factors increasing extracellular fluid volume, those causing vasoconstriction, and those influencing cardiac output (Figure 2-1). This mechanistic approach is useful in understanding the pathogenesis and treatment of hypertension (see Chapters 5 through 8) and in providing some degree of insight into the different manifestations, consequences, and complications of elevated blood pressure.

Factors That Influence Extracellular Fluid Volume

Fluid composes 55% to 60% of total body weight; 40% of that fluid is in the extracellular compartment and the rest is intracellular. The major constituent of extracellular fluid is sodium, which accounts for more than 90% of the osmotic effect in this fluid compartment. The extracellu-

Table 2-1: Factors That Influence Extracellular Fluid Volume

A. Sodium Intake

B. Vascular Factors:	C. Hormone Factors:
glomerular filtration rate	angiotensin II (AT_1)
vascular resistance	norepinephrine (α)
glomerular capillary pressure	kinins
endothelin	prostaglandins
nitric oxide	adenosine
vasopressin	atrial natriuretic factor
	aldosterone

lar compartment can be further separated into interstitial fluid and circulating plasma volume. Exchange between interstitial and plasma volume components is influenced by the hydrostatic and osmotic pressures of each. In general, blood pressure correlates more closely with plasma volume in healthy subjects but with interstitial fluid in hypertensive patients. Most studies that have measured plasma volume in hypertensives have failed to find an elevation in absolute terms. Nonetheless, this apparently 'normal' plasma volume in hypertension may actually be inappropriate. Patients with hypertension have an increase in vascular resistance and vasoconstriction as well as a decrease in compliance and elasticity of the vasculature and rarefaction of capillary and tertiary arteriolar structures. Therefore, the plasma volume can be construed to be disproportionately increased for the reduced vascular capacity.

What factors influence extracellular fluid balance? The major factors are summarized in Table 2-1. Obviously, a major determinant is the ability of the kidneys to excrete salt as the major osmolyte and, therefore, the water that follows through passive diffusion. The kidneys act selectively, serving as more than mere filters because sodium is a major determinant of fluid balance and nutrient exchange. The active and important role of the kidneys in handling sodium results from the very large concentration gradient for sodium between extracellular (135 to 145 mmoL) and intracellular (3 to 30 mmoL) compartments. The cells are protected against rupture that could result from the intrusion of sodium and the passive diffusion of water. This protection is provided by a variety of active, energy-dependent systems or 'pumps,' and ionic exchange factors that extrude sodium against this large concentration gradient.[2]

Recent evidence indicates that patients with hypertension have abnormalities in some of these systems, including some genetic abnormalities. One such system, sodium-lithium countertransport, is linked to the pathogenesis of hypertension, presumably by permitting an increase in the intracellular sodium concentration that is observed in some patients. According to this hypothesis, the increased sodium content of vascular tissue in some way enhances the pressor response to ambient factors that influence vascular tone. Another candidate of the cellular transport system implicated in hypertension is the sodium-hydrogen ion exchanger. It is hypothesized that an abnormality of this system could promote changes in intracellular pH that could then trigger other events and culminate in increased vascular tone. Recent evidence implicates the involvement of intracellular calcium concentration in the ionic shifts between intracellular and extracellular compartments, and in the response of vascular tissue to contractile and relaxant stimuli.[3] Both current and future studies will likely elucidate the role of these and other systems involved in maintaining cellular ionic equilibrium in the pathogenesis and maintenance of hypertension.

Apart from the intracellular mechanisms for ion transport, the kidneys influence sodium and water balance in a variety of ways.[1] Approximately one fourth of cardiac output is committed to the delivery of blood to the kidneys (renal blood flow). Blood is filtered by the kidneys with selective reabsorption of nutrients and other requisite plasma components and excretion of waste products. A variety of influences on reabsorption and excretion occur at different sites along the nephron. Over a 24-hour period, the healthy kidney produces approximately 180 L of filtrate from the blood it receives, 99% of which is subsequently reabsorbed, and only about 1% of which is excreted in the urine. Thus, it is apparent that one of the major determinants of extracellular fluid volume is the glomerular filtration rate (GFR). Glomerular filtration rate is influenced by cardiac output, the patency of the renal arteries and arterioles, and the number and functional integrity of filtering units (glomeruli and nephrons). A reduction in glomeruli or nephrons can occur as the result of currently unidentified congenital factors associated with reduced birth weight.[4]

In addition, intrinsic renal disease that involves the glomerulus and/or nephron, or that is induced by hemodynamic changes, such as glomerular hyperfiltration or increased hydrostatic pressure, can also reduce the filtering efficiency of the kidneys. An example of this is in diabetes mellitus, where hyperfiltration and possibly glomerular injury from metabolic factors, such as elevated glucose levels and their by-products, or lipid and lipoprotein abnormalities that often accompany diabetes, lead to glomerulosclerosis and obliteration of glomeruli.[5] These changes further influence GFR and glomerular pressure as well as contribute to tubular damage. This increases the load on the remaining glomeruli and accelerates the destruction of glomeruli and nephrons, which lead to a vicious circle that ultimately produces renal failure. Recent evidence suggests that increased dietary protein intake can also exacerbate such disease-related impairments of renal function and that protein restriction can slow the progression of renal impairment in some subjects.[6]

The tone and pressure of the renal vasculature, from the main renal arteries to the arterioles that supply and drain the glomerulus, modulate glomerular and nephron function by altering both blood flow and pressure. Some researchers have proposed that circulating vasoactive substances can influence renal function by modulating changes in glomerular capillary pressure.[7] This may be related to the differential effects of angiotensin II, norepinephrine, and other vasoactive substances on the efferent and afferent arterioles of the glomerulus. Therefore, an increase in sympathetic tone or activity would preferentially constrict the afferent arteriole and reduce glomerular capillary blood flow and pressure. It is known that this is mediated by α-adrenergic receptors and theoretically could be prevented or remedied by drugs that induce α-adrenergic receptor blockade. In addition, vasoconstriction of the afferent vessel may be modulated by prostaglandins and by vasodilatory effects exerted at this level by bradykinin and nitric oxide.

An increase in the activity of the renin-angiotensin system plays a relatively greater role in inducing constriction of the efferent arteriole and, therefore, in raising glomerular capillary pressure. This is opposed by the vasodilatory effect of nitric oxide, which may be reduced in hypertension. This concept led to the development of specific therapeutic strategies, as in diabetic nephropathy, where angiotensin-converting enzyme (ACE) inhibitors have reduced the development or progression of renal disease.[8] It is thought that diabetic nephropathy progresses from glomerular hyperfiltration through stages of increased glomerular capillary pressure, glomerulosclerosis, and then progressive obliteration of glomeruli and nephrons because of the added burden on the remaining functioning glomeruli and nephrons. One hypothesis is that the initial abnormalities of increased glomerular capillary pressure and hyperfiltration are influenced by increased levels of angiotensin II. Thus, the blunting of this effect of the renin-angiotensin system by ACE inhibitors and, at least theoretically, by angiotensin II-receptor antagonists, could reduce this hemodynamic aberration and slow the progression of diabetic nephropathy. This will likely be demonstrated with the results of several ongoing studies involving angiotensin (AT_1) receptor blockers.

The renal hemodynamic situation is further complicated by the fact that both norepinephrine and angiotensin II can stimulate the release of prostaglandins that can have multiple effects on the renal vasculature and on glomerular function. Kinins and nitric oxide also influence the vasodilatory responses of the arterioles and further modulate renal hemodynamics. A variety of circulating or locally produced humoral factors can influence reabsorption of sodium and/or water at both the proximal and more distal parts of the nephron. Examples of such circulating substances include the adrenal mineralocorticoid aldosterone, which causes sodium reabsorption at the collecting system of the kidneys in exchange for potassium and hydrogen ions; vasopressin, which influences water excretion; and atrial natriuretic peptide, which similarly influences sodium and water excretion. All three of these substances affect vascular tone.

The latter two hormones are apparently regulated by single factors. Plasma osmolality typically controls vasopressin release; atrial stretch, which is a reflection of extracellular fluid volume status, determines atrial natriuretic peptide release. However, in the case of aldosterone, multiple stimuli are recognized.

The primary stimulus for aldosterone production is angiotensin II, the product of the renin system, which is stimulated by a perceived decrease in macula densa sodium concentration or by pressure at the level of the juxtaglomerular apparatus of the kidneys. In addition, angiotensin II may have a direct effect on sodium reabsorption, as discussed below. A second stimulus for aldosterone release, active when the renin system is suppressed, is adrenocorticotrophic hormone from the pituitary gland. An additional modulating influence is serum potassium, which is influenced by the level of aldosterone. Recently, several other steroid effects have been shown to influence sodium handling by the kidneys.

When aldosterone, the prototype mineralocorticoid, occupies its renal receptor, it causes renal sodium reabsorption and induces expansion of extracellular fluid volume. This receptor also recognizes other steroids with a chemical structure similar to aldosterone, such as cortisol. It has always been puzzling that cortisol, which normally circulates in plasma in a concentration 1,000 times higher than that of aldosterone and which has equal affinity for the mineralocorticoid receptor in vitro, does not typically have a significant impact on renal sodium reabsorption. We have recently learned that the reason for this inability of cortisol to occupy the mineralocorticoid receptor under normal circumstances is that cortisol is made inactive by conversion to cortisone by the enzyme 11β-hydroxysteroid dehydrogenase.[9] The mineralocorticoid receptor has a much lower affinity for cortisone. This recent observation helped to explain several forms of hypertension that resemble primary aldosteronism (see Chapter 4), hence the name of apparent mineralocorticoid excess syndrome. Two exogenous agents, licorice and carbenoxolone, competitively inhibit 11β-hydroxysteroid dehydrogenase and, thus, impair the cortisol-to-cortisone conversion and permit activation of the renal mineralocorticoid receptor by cortisol.[9] In addition, genetic abnormalities of steroid synthesis and metabolism, discussed in the section dealing with primary aldosteronism (see Chapter 4), can also produce steroids that promote renal sodium retention and extracellular volume expansion.

In addition to stimulating aldosterone production, angiotensin II can also directly influence sodium and water reabsorption either by reducing renal blood flow as a result of its hemodynamic effect to induce efferent arteriolar vasoconstriction, or by its ability to increase tubular sodium ion transport.

Drugs that influence the renin-angiotensin-aldosterone system in a variety of ways include aldosterone antagonists, β-adrenergic blocking agents, ACE inhibitors, angiotensin II receptor blockers (ARBs), and renin inhibitors. These drugs have markedly enhanced the understanding of the role of various components of this system in human physiology and in the pathophysiology and treatment of hypertension and other disorders. Some of these insights are discussed in more detail in the chapters dealing with antihypertensive drug therapy (see Chapters 6 through 8).

A variety of endothelial components produce substances or serve as targets for factors that can alter vascular behavior, renal blood flow, and glomerular filtration rate, and also directly influence tubular function. As examples, vasoactive prostaglandins, endothelial-derived relaxing factor (nitric oxide), adenosine, and bradykinin have all been shown to influence renal hemodynamics and/or sodium handling by the kidneys. New information about the roles of these factors in human hypertension will provide additional useful therapeutic approaches in the future.

Systemic Vascular Resistance

An increase in peripheral vascular resistance is a typical feature of hypertension. There is extensive debate about whether this is a primary event or one that develops as part of the vascular adaptation to blood pressure elevation itself, a process referred to as vascular remodeling. Understanding of blood vessel physiology has progressed from an initial concept of the vasculature as a simple conduit for blood and oxygen with simplistic contractile and relaxant activity. We now recognize the blood vessel as a complex vascular organ with smooth muscle layers that have dynamic responses, and the endothelium as an endo-

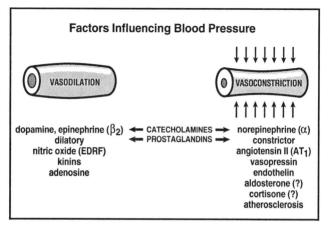

Figure 2-2: Factors that influence blood pressure.

crine, paracrine, and autocrine organ with receptors for a variety of vasoactive substances. This enhanced understanding of vascular biology has provided an explanation for why some antihypertensive drugs, which were developed empirically with little or no understanding of how they worked, lower blood pressure. For example, sodium nitroprusside, which is a relaxant of vascular smooth muscle, was used in the treatment of hypertension long before the sophisticated interplay of endothelium and vascular smooth muscle was recognized.

The sympathetic nervous system has long been recognized as a participant in elevated blood pressure in many individuals. Early observations of catecholamine-induced vasoconstriction led to the recognition that blood vessels respond in different ways to specific catecholamine agonists. Elucidation of α-adrenergic, β-adrenergic, and dopaminergic receptor subtypes enhanced our understanding of circulatory dynamics. Blockers of these receptors provided approaches to the treatment of a variety of disorders, including hypertension, discussed in detail in Chapters 5 through 7. Systemic vascular resistance is determined by the net effect of several factors acting on the blood vessel, as depicted in Figure 2-2.

The role of the kidneys in influencing blood pressure, independent of renal handling of sodium and water, has been recognized for 100 years.[10] Tigerstedt and Bergman demonstrated that injection of a kidney extract from one animal into the circulation of another anephric animal caused an immediate and dramatic increase in arterial pressure. During the 1920s, Goldblatt and Haas demonstrated that a reduction in blood flow to the kidneys of dogs produced an increase in blood pressure. Two subsequent studies done simultaneously in the 1940s by Helmer and Page, and by Fasciolo and Braun-Menendez, demonstrated that the pressor substance from the kidneys, renin, acted by producing a vasoconstrictor peptide they jointly named angiotensin, using the separate names that each group had given this substance—angiotonin and hypertensin. Thus, knowledge of the renin-angiotensin system evolved. This system has been extensively investigated and new aspects of its physiology continue to be elucidated.

Angiotensin II is one of the most potent vasoconstrictors known. It also acts to induce growth of vascular smooth muscle and contributes to vascular remodeling. In addition, angiotensin II affects cardiac myocyte growth and contractility, actions that contribute to its role in left ventricular hypertrophy. This complex network of factors provides a rich substrate for pharmacologic manipulation and for the development of new therapeutic approaches, not only in hypertension, but also in a variety of cardiovascular and related disorders. For example, the use of β-adrenergic-blocking agents in the treatment of hypertension was at least partially derived from the observations that renin release from the kidneys required intact renal β-adrenergic receptor activity. Therefore, β-blocking drugs prevent renin release and limit angiotensin-dependent blood pressure increases. Although this is not the only ac-

Table 2-2: Factors That Influence Cardiac Output

A. Extracellular Fluid Volume

B. Heart Rate	**C. Contractility**
Catecholamines (β_1)	Catecholamines (α, β_1)
Vagal tone	Angiotensin II (AT_1)

tion of β-blockers that contributes to the blood pressure-lowering effects (see Cardiac Output section), it was one of the early factors used to explain these effects.

The development of ACE inhibitors capable of preventing the conversion of the initial product of renin's action on its substrate, angiotensin I, to the active peptide, angiotensin II, added another dimension to the understanding of the role of this system in human physiology and disease and a new approach to the treatment of many disorders. The availability of ARBs has further enriched therapeutic choices, and investigative studies of renin inhibitors may provide additional useful therapies.

In addition to catecholamines and the renin-angiotensin system, other vasoconstrictive factors have been identified. These include vasopressin, the prostaglandins with constrictor activities, and endothelin, which is produced locally by the endothelium itself. Vascular tone and resistance can also be modulated by factors that cause vasodilation. Circulating or local levels of dopamine, vasodilatory prostaglandins, atrial natriuretic factor, local kinins, adenosine, and the endothelium-derived relaxing factor, nitric oxide, are all involved in vascular physiology and blood pressure control. Moreover, many of the vasoactive factors have interactions with other components that may modulate their effects. The future should bring new therapeutic approaches directed toward these components as well.

Cardiac Output

The third component of blood pressure control, cardiac output, is largely influenced by factors that also influence extracellular fluid volume and vascular resistance (Table 2-2). Circulating blood volume is an obvious component of cardiac output. Additionally, heart rate and myocardial contractility are major determinants. Substantial evidence from observational and epidemiologic studies indicates that essential hypertension has its origins in increased sympathetic nervous system activity and increased cardiac output. The Tecumseh study, a prospective, community-based, long-term observational study, demonstrated that initially normotensive subjects who developed hypertension could be identified before the rise in their blood pressure by increased pulse rate, increased plasma norepinephrine levels, and insulin resistance, all manifestations of enhanced sympathetic nervous system activity and/or responsiveness.[11] Similarly, young men with borderline hypertension had resting tachycardia and a hyperdynamic chest wall on physical examination, which reflected increased sympathetic nervous system activity. The explanation of the pathophysiologic events leading to the development of essential hypertension in some subjects begins with this sympathetically mediated increase in cardiac output. Then, after a period of blood pressure elevation, vascular adaptation and remodeling lead to an increase in vascular resistance and a decrease in elasticity and compliance of the capacitance circuit. This produces relative volume excess in the absence of a demonstrably increased total extracellular fluid volume compartment.

Heart rate can also be influenced by the interplay of β_1-adrenergic receptor stimulation and vagal tone. Thus, drugs that influence these components, such as β_1-adrenergic receptor blockers and vagolytic agents, influence cardiac output. Myocardial contractility can also be influenced by a variety of factors. These include catecholamines that act through the α-receptor mechanism and angiotensin II, which apparently has specific actions on myocardial tissue. Beta-adrenergic receptor blockers can influence blood pressure by reducing heart rate and decreasing myocardial contractility.

References

1. Guyton AC, Hall JE, Coleman TG, et al: The dominant role of the kidneys in long-term arterial pressure regulation in normal and hypertensive states. In: Laragh JH, Brenner, BM, eds. *Hypertension: Pathophysiology, Diagnosis, and Management*, 2nd ed. New York, Raven Press, 1995, pp 1311-1326.

2. Aviv A: The lymphocyte Na+/H+ antiport and its activation by increased NaCl intake: the link with salt sensitivity and cellular Ca^2+ regulation. *Eur J Clin Invest* 1994;24:525-528.

3. Aviv A: Cytosolic Ca^2, Na+/H+ antiport, protein kinase C trio in essential hypertension. *Am J Hypertens* 1994;7:205-212.

4. Kimura G, Frem GJ, Brenner BM: Renal mechanisms of salt sensitivity in hypertension. *Curr Opin Nephrol Hypertens* 1994;3:1-12.

5. National High Blood Pressure Education Program Working Group Report on Hypertension in Diabetes. *Hypertension* 1994;23:145-158.

6. Klahr S, Levey AS, Beck GJ, et al: The effects of dietary protein restriction and blood pressure control on the progression of chronic renal disease. *N Engl J Med* 1994;330:877-884.

7. Hall JE, Guyton AC, Brands MW: Control of sodium excretion and arterial pressure by intrarenal mechanisms and the renin-angiotensin system. In: Laragh JH, Brenner BM, eds. *Hypertension: Pathophysiology, Diagnosis, and Management*, 2nd ed. New York, Raven Press, 1995, pp 1451-1475.

8. Lewis EJ, Hunsicker LG, Bain RP, et al: The effect of angiotensin-converting enzyme inhibition on diabetic nephropathy. *N Engl J Med* 1993;329:1456-1462.

9. Edwards C, Walker B: Cortisol and hypertension: what was not so apparent about 'apparent mineralocorticoid excess.' *J Lab Clin Med* 1993;122:632-635.

10. Sealey JE, Laragh JH: The renin-angiotensin-aldosterone system for normal regulation of blood pressure and sodium and

potassium homeostasis. In: Laragh JH, Brenner BM, eds. *Hypertension: Pathophysiology, Diagnosis, and Management*, 2nd ed. New York, Raven Press, 1995, pp 1763-1796.

11. Julius S, Mejia A, Jones K, et al: 'White coat' versus 'sustained' borderline hypertension in Tecumseh, Michigan. *Hypertension* 1990;16:617-623.

Chapter 3

Evaluation of Primary or Essential Hypertension

Before an extensive and expensive evaluation of hypertension is initiated, a patient should demonstrate a persistent elevation of blood pressure. Unless this elevation is severe or there is evidence of end-organ involvement, this demonstration typically requires documentation of blood pressure elevation in excess of 140/90 mm Hg (or greater than 140 systolic in the case of isolated systolic hypertension) on at least two separate occasions, separated by several days or weeks. In some individuals, taking blood pressure in the hospital, clinic, or office can be associated with a higher blood pressure reading than when blood pressure is measured in a different environment. This is referred to as the *white coat* effect.[1] This effect is not entirely innocuous because it has been associated with evidence of end-organ disease, particularly left ventricular enlargement. This finding implies that the medical setting is not the only environment capable of inducing an excessive increase in blood pressure in such individuals.

The possibility that blood pressure elevation only occurs in the office or clinic setting can be evaluated further by 24-hour ambulatory blood pressure monitoring, using an automated device capable of taking blood pressure at predetermined intervals during a 24-hour to 48-hour period and storing the data for subsequent analysis. Alternatively, the use of a home blood pressure cuff, with proper instructions for accurate use, can provide additional information on which to base therapeutic decisions. If this option is chosen, several considerations can enhance its value. It is important that the blood pressure measurement be accurate (see Chapter 1), that the equipment be calibrated at least every 6 months, that the blood pressure cuff be the appropriate size for arm circumference, that the patient be relaxed, that the room or environment not be cold, and that the patient's arm be at heart level.

Exogenous Causes of Elevated Blood Pressure

Exogenous factors should be considered when evaluating the patient with hypertension. For example, severe anxiety or pain can cause an elevated blood pressure, as can the use of sympathomimetic agents such as nasal sprays, decongestants, and appetite suppressants. 'Street' or recreational drugs such as amphetamines and cocaine represent other exogenous causes of hypertension. Commonly prescribed and over-the-counter agents such as nonsteroidal anti-inflammatory drugs (NSAIDs) can have a pressor effect and should be considered when evaluating a patient with evidence of recent blood pressure elevation. The use of corticosteroids for the treatment of a variety of disorders or anabolic steroids for muscle building can also contribute to blood pressure elevation. The treatment for transplant rejection that includes cyclosporine and corticosteroids can be associated with elevation of blood pressure. Habitual alcohol consumption in excess of 2 to 3 oz a day can raise blood pressure.[2] In addition, increased dietary intake of sodium or a decreased intake of potassium or calcium may be associated with the development of hypertension in susceptible individuals. This is discussed in detail in Chapter 5.

Twenty to 30 years ago, oral contraceptives constituted a major identifiable cause of hypertension,[3] but current preparations have a reduced estrogen content and have thus become a less frequent contributor to elevated blood pressure. On the other hand, the striking increase in use of estrogens for the treatment of menopausal symptoms and for the prevention of osteoporosis has contributed to hypertension in some older women. This effect appears to be dose dependent, and occurs more often at doses of conjugated estrogen greater than 0.625 mg/d (or its equivalence). When hypertension is documented in a woman receiving estrogen, a trial of estrogen withdrawal is often justified to observe the effect on blood pressure. However, several months of estrogen withdrawal may be required before the maximal effects on blood pressure are observed. Obviously, the benefits of estrogen therapy must be considered for such an individual and balanced against the risks associated with blood pressure elevation and the difficulty associated with maintaining blood pressure control during hormone replacement therapy.

As mentioned in Chapter 2, licorice inhibits the effect of 11β-hydroxysteroid dehydrogenase, which permits cortisol to occupy the mineralocorticoid receptor and thus promotes salt and water retention by the kidneys and volume expansion. Rarely, individuals who consistently ingest large amounts (15 g to 20 g) of licorice candy develop hypertension and the manifestations of mineralocorticoid excess.

History

After confirming elevated blood pressure and asking the patient about potential exogenous causes, the clinician should perform a comprehensive history and physical examination. The goals are to assess evidence of end-organ disease, to evaluate the likelihood of a secondary form of hypertension, and to identify other cardiovascular disease risk factors and disorders that require attention and that may influence the choice of treatment.

Both the patient and the physician or health-care provider must recognize that hypertension is generally asymptomatic, so that specific symptoms are unusual. Asking the patient about the occurrence of headaches is appropriate, including their nature, frequency, severity, and any recent changes. Many patients believe that headaches are a manifestation of elevated blood pressure and that they can 'tell' if blood pressure is elevated by the presence of a headache. There is no scientific confirmation of this belief because the frequency of headache is no different in hypertensives than in normotensive subjects. More likely, some antihypertensive medications produce headache in some individuals. However, when blood pressure elevation is severe, headache may be a manifestation of hypertensive encephalopathy.

Other manifestations of hypertensive central nervous system involvement include blurred vision and any of a number of neurologic symptoms that range from paresthesias to coma. Occasionally, the initial recognition of elevated blood pressure results from a routine ophthalmologic examination when the presence of hypertensive retinopathy is noted and prompts a referral to a primary care provider for additional evaluation and treatment. A history of thyroid disorders and treatment is also important because hypertension may occur with either hyperthyroidism or hypothyroidism. The former is more often associated with a greater increase in systolic pressure, whereas diastolic elevation is more typically found in hypothyroidism.

The clinician must investigate any findings or symptoms of cardiovascular disease, such as congenital problems, angina, or congestive heart failure. Such symptoms may represent the presence of heart disease and may alter the therapeutic choices for blood pressure control. Clues should be sought about other cardiovascular disease risk factors such as diabetes mellitus, dyslipidemia, left ventricular hypertrophy, and tobacco use. A history of pulmonary disease or asthma should be ascertained because this may also influence therapeutic decisions, such as avoidance of β-adrenergic receptor-blocking agents or angiotensin-converting enzyme (ACE) inhibitors. Sleep disorders or snoring should also be evaluated because sleep apnea is often associated with hypertension and can be treated with a variety of approaches.[4]

Gastrointestinal symptoms should be evaluated because treatment (eg, anticholinergics, fiber, stool softeners) may interfere with the efficacy of antihypertensive therapy. Thus, the timing of administration of various therapies becomes important. In addition, blood pressure treatment can cause or worsen some gastrointestinal symptoms, such as nausea, esophagogastritis, or constipation. Because the kidneys are intimately involved in blood pressure control, a detailed evaluation of genitourinary symptoms is important. Information about renal stones, infections, hematuria, proteinuria, polyuria, and nocturia are all appropriate and may provide clues about the presence of renal disease. A history of persistent nocturia in men may infer prostatic disease. Moreover, treatment with peripheral α_1-adrenergic receptor-blocking agents such as prazosin (Minipress®), terazosin (Hytrin®), or doxazosin (Cardura®) may then be considered for both the elevated blood pressure and the symptoms of prostatism. Obtaining a history of sexual function is appropriate because impairment is often observed in patients with hypertension and because some antihypertensive agents may exacerbate or induce such problems. Evaluation of edema and peripheral vascular disease symptoms is also important.

Information concerning alcohol consumption and diet, and a history of both over-the-counter and prescription drug use, should be obtained. Information about elevated blood pressure readings and any drug treatment should also be noted, with consideration of both the blood pressure response to medications and the occurrence of side effects.

Physical Examination

Observation of body habitus ('apple' or 'pear' shape), measurement of body weight, and examination of facial appearance and affect are appropriate. On initial evaluation,

Table 3-1: Recommended Laboratory Evaluation of Primary ('Essential') Hypertension

Routine	Optional
Urine analysis	Creatinine clearance
Complete blood count	Urinary protein excretion
Fasting glucose	Echocardiogram
Lipid profile (including HDL, total cholesterol, and triglycerides)	
Electrolytes and calcium	
Blood urea nitrogen and creatinine	
Uric acid	
Electrocardiogram	

the blood pressure should be measured in both arms and in one leg. A marked discrepancy in blood pressure between the arms suggests an obstructive vascular lesion. When co-arctation of the aorta is present, the blood pressure in the legs is substantially lower than that in the arms. Pulse rate should also be measured while the patient is sitting. To identify orthostatic hypotension, blood pressure should first be measured after a few minutes of recumbency and then after 2 minutes of standing. This is particularly important in older individuals, in diabetics, and in those taking antihypertensive therapy.

An evaluation of neurologic status is appropriate. A careful ophthalmologic evaluation, including retinoscopy, is important. The thyroid should be evaluated. The chest, lungs, and heart should be examined to identify the presence of congestive heart failure, cardiac enlargement, hypertrophy, arrhythmias, or murmurs. The abdominal examination should include palpation of abdominal organs

37

and kidneys, and careful auscultation in the midepigastric areas, flanks, and femoral arteries for the presence of a bruit signaling vascular disease. The peripheral pulses should be examined and the presence of peripheral edema noted. Deep tendon reflexes and sensory evaluation should also be performed.

Laboratory Evaluation

The laboratory evaluation of patients *not* suspected of having a secondary form of hypertension has three goals: (1) assessment of the degree of end-organ involvement; (2) identification of other cardiovascular disease risk factors, both of which permit stratification for therapeutic decision making; and (3) establishment of a baseline from which to evaluate progression of end-organ disease and the effect of drug therapy. The basic components of this evaluation are outlined in Table 3-1. A routine urine analysis should be performed to identify cellular elements, protein, or glucose. Also routine are a complete blood count, fasting blood sugar, a lipid profile that includes triglycerides, total cholesterol, and high-density lipoprotein (HDL), electrolytes, blood urea nitrogen (BUN), creatinine clearance, calcium, and uric acid. Automated chemistry profiles often include most or all of these components at reduced cost. A more accurate measure of renal function than simple blood tests includes an endogenous 24-hour creatinine clearance study and, if indicated, 24-hour urinary protein excretion.

An electrocardiogram is also routinely recommended to evaluate the possibility of coronary artery disease, arrhythmias, or left ventricular hypertrophy, as well as to provide a baseline for future evaluation. Considerable debate exists regarding the inclusion of an echocardiogram for the routine evaluation of an uncomplicated asymptomatic patient with hypertension. Although echocardiography is a more sensitive tool for identifying left ventricular hypertrophy in hypertension and can provide information about left ventricular and valvular function, its expense for routine use causes reticence. Several ongoing studies are examining the significance of left ventricular hypertrophy in predicting outcome in treated hypertension. The results of these studies, the comparison of various criteria for its identification, and the evolution of less expensive echocardiographic techniques may settle these issues in the future.

References

1.   Pickering TG, James GD, Boddie C, et al: How common is white coat hypertension? *JAMA* 1988;259:225-228.

2.   Maheswaran R, Gill JS, Davies P, et al: High blood pressure due to alcohol: a rapidly reversible effect. *Hypertension* 1991; 17:787-792.

3.   Weinberger MH, Collins RD, Dowdy AJ, et al: Hypertension induced by oral contraceptives containing estrogen and gestagen. *Ann Intern Med* 1969;71:891-902.

4.   Askenasy JJ, Tanne D: The inter-relationship between sleep apnea syndrome and hypertension. *Isr J Med Sci* 1995;31: 561-567.

Chapter 4

Evaluation for Secondary Forms of Hypertension

P atients who are more likely to have a secondary form of hypertension include those who were young when found to have elevated pressure or those whose rise in blood pressure is sudden or marked. Primary hypertension typically occurs when the patient is in the 40s and 50s and demonstrates a gradual and progressive course. Severe or refractory hypertension may also be a clue to an underlying identifiable etiology.

History

In addition to the history information outlined in Chapter 3, clinicians should consider specific questions about signs and symptoms of secondary forms of hypertension. To provide a systematic approach to such inquiry, it is useful to be aware of the most common secondary causes of elevated blood pressure (Table 4-1).

Inquiry into the presence of symptoms of renal disease may provide a clue about this secondary cause of hypertension. Rarely, patients with renal vascular hypertension may report episodes of flank pain, but this is more common with renal parenchymal disease or kidney stones. A history of flank trauma should prompt consideration of perinephritis ('Page' kidney) resulting from hemorrhage into the renal capsule.[1]

Table 4-1: Common Forms of Secondary Hypertension

- Renal parenchymal disease
- Renal vascular hypertension
- Primary aldosteronism
- Pheochromocytoma
- Cushing's syndrome
- Hyperthyroidism or hypothyroidism
- Collagen vascular disease
- Perinephritis ('Page' kidney)

Patients with primary aldosteronism often have muscle weakness and cramps related to associated electrolyte abnormalities (hypokalemia and hypomagnesemia). Severe headaches and nocturia are also common in such patients. Because some forms of primary aldosteronism are genetically mediated, a familial incidence of hypertension may be observed.

Although episodic hypertension may occur in patients with pheochromocytoma, it is present in only 15% to 20% of cases, with most patients having fixed hypertension.[2] Tremors are not typical with this adrenal tumor, nor is flushing. In contrast, pallor, coldness of the extremities, and tachycardia are more usual manifestations of the excessive catecholamine production.[2] Pheochromocytoma may be familial, typically as part of a multiple endocrine neoplasia syndrome, and may be associated with neurofibromas and cafe-au-lait skin lesions.

The symptoms of thyroid disease are varied and nonspecific. Hyperthyroidism may be suggested by weight loss, diarrhea, tachycardia, hair changes, and heat intolerance. Symptoms of hypothyroidism include slow speech, coldness, thick skin, brittle hair, and constipation. Women may note alterations in menstrual cycle. In older patients, the typical manifestations of hyperthyroidism, which are largely mediated by catecholamines, may be masked so that these patients may present with atrial fibrillation, other cardiac arrhythmias, or cardiac symptoms.

Physical Examination

Patients with advanced renal disease often have distinct skin and breath changes. Patients with primary aldosteronism may develop tetanic muscle cramps when the blood pressure cuff is inflated (Trousseau's sign). Despite elevation of blood pressure that is often severe and long standing, patients with primary aldosteronism typically have minimal eyeground changes. This finding may also be present in essential (or primary) hypertension of the 'low-renin' subgroup, which suggests that hypertensive retinopathy may require increased levels of vasoconstrictor peptides such as angiotensin II or catecholamines as well as elevated blood pressure. Evidence to support this concept is derived from the frequent reports of severe hypertensive retinopathy in patients with renal vascular hypertension or pheochromocytoma. In the latter, neurofibromas, which are small, fluctuant, nontender nodules distributed primarily over the trunk, may be found. Skin lesions (cafe-au-lait spots) are also seen in some patients with pheochromocytoma.

Cushing's syndrome may be suggested by the findings of a rounded facial appearance ('moon' facies), facial plethora, prominent cervical fat pads, a 'buffalo hump' produced by increased posterior cervical fat deposition, truncal obesity with thin extremities, and purple skin striae on the abdominal wall and thighs. Patients with collagen vascular disease may have a malar skin rash, petechiae, or joint abnormalities that may provide a clue to the underlying disorder. Typically, hypertension in patients with collagen vascular disease is associated with renal involvement.

Thyroid disorders are associated with a variety of physical findings. In hyperthyroidism, a host of eye abnormalities may occur, most often exophthalmos, and also lid lag on upward gaze and a fine tremor of the hands. Thyroid enlargement is often but not invariably present. Fine, silky hair texture is also common. With hypothyroidism, dry or cracked skin may occur. A brawny form of edema ('myxedema') may be seen over the shins. The mucinous texture of myxedema makes it difficult to 'pit,' which helps to differentiate it from dependent edema caused by fluid accumulation.

About half of patients with renal vascular hypertension have a *continuous* (as opposed to systolic only) abdominal bruit.[3] This is usually heard best in the midepigastrium and may require pressure on the head of the stethoscope to hear. In thin individuals, the bruit may be more pronounced over the flanks or even the vertebrae. The bruit may radiate laterally from the midepigastrium. Whereas a systolic abdominal bruit is common in patients both with and without hypertension and thus has no pathognomonic significance for renal vascular disease, the presence of a *continuous* abdominal bruit (systolic-diastolic) in a patient with hypertension is almost always associated with a functionally significant renal artery lesion. Unfortunately, the absence of such a bruit does not rule out the presence of renal vascular disease.[3]

Laboratory Evaluation

Appropriate evaluation of the various secondary forms of hypertension is separated into consideration of screening tests, diagnostic procedures, localization techniques, and therapeutic approaches for each of the more common of these disorders.

Renal Vascular Hypertension

The definitive procedure for the identification of renal vascular lesions is a renal arteriogram. Because of this procedure's expense and risks, alternative screening tests are generally tried first. The most frequently used is the radioisotopic renal scan, particularly in combination with acute administration of an angiotensin-converting enzyme (ACE) inhibitor.[4] A brief review of the pathophysiology of renal vascular disease makes the rationale for this approach more understandable. In the presence of a functionally significant renal arterial lesion, a reduction in renal blood flow and pressure to the involved kidney is recognized by the juxtaglomerular apparatus. This hemodynamic change stimulates the renin-angiotensin system in an attempt to increase renal blood flow and pressure. The increased pressure induced by the increase in renin and angiotensin in the systemic circulation, however, is not effectively transmitted to the involved kidney because of the obstructive arterial lesion. Thus, the increase in renin and angiotensin persists. Within the involved kidney, the reduction in flow and pressure seen by the glomerulus would soon cause glomerular failure were it not for the local effect of angiotensin II, which induces preferential efferent arteriolar constriction and thereby increases glomerular capillary pressure and maintains the pressure required to sustain glomerular filtration.

When an isotope that is cleared by the kidney is administered intravenously to a patient with renal vascular hypertension involving one kidney, the involved kidney is slower to receive the isotope than the uninvolved kidney because of the reduction in flow and pressure. The pattern of excretion of the isotope is also delayed in the involved kidney because of the reduction in glomerular flow and pressure. This discrepancy in the appearance and excretion of the isotope between the involved and uninvolved kidney is accentuated when an ACE inhibitor is administered. The ACE inhibitor decreases angiotensin II production and thus effectively removes the drive for glomerular filtration in the involved kidney: the efferent arteriolar constriction induced by angiotensin II.[4] Most studies have used relatively short-acting ACE inhibitors for this purpose, such as captopril (Capoten®) or enalapril (Vasotec®). The latter is available in both intravenous and oral forms. The angiotensin II receptor blockers (ARBs) may prove to be as effective as ACE inhibitors in enhancing this mode of detecting renal vascular hypertension.

Renal vascular disease is often bilateral, which may diminish the disparity in renal blood flow and function seen on a scan. However, in most cases of bilateral disease, one side is more significantly involved than the other, and both kidneys usually show a delayed pattern of isotope accumulation and excretion, which enables identification of an abnormality by an experienced reviewer. The renal isotopic scan has replaced the intravenous pyelogram as the screening test of choice for renal vascular hypertension because of the latter's higher rate of false-negative and false-positive results.[4]

After a positive isotopic scan is observed, the diagnosis of renal vascular hypertension requires the demonstration of a significant renal arterial lesion. Renal arteriography is typically used for this purpose. Using computer enhancement of the vasculature, digitized vascular imaging procedures have recently enabled arterial imaging with less contrast administration than is required for conventional arteriography.[5] The anatomic definition of an obstructive lesion of the renal vasculature alone in a hypertensive patient is not sufficient evidence that the lesion is responsible for the blood pressure elevation. The ultimate proof of the functional significance of a renal arterial lesion is, obviously, the improvement or cure of hypertension after successful revascularization. However, some observations strongly support the functional significance of lesions and aid in the decision about intervention. The presence of a continuous abdominal bruit, as mentioned, is a helpful sign.[3] A clear-cut alteration in renal blood flow after administration of an ACE inhibitor is another physiologic clue.[4] A poststenotic dilatation on arteriography strongly suggests a hemodynamically significant lesion. Some radiologists measure intra-arterial pressure gradients proximal and distal to the stenotic lesion during performance of arteriography, which provides direct quantitative evidence of the degree of stenosis.

Because renal vascular hypertension is induced by the inappropriate release of renin by the involved kidney (or the more-involved kidney in the case of bilateral renal arterial disease), measurement of renal venous renin content to compare the concentration in both kidneys *and* the inferior vena cava is still one of the best predictors of a beneficial response to intervention.[3] However, the value of renal venous renin studies requires careful attention to several issues. First, the patient should be withdrawn from agents that suppress renin release, because these could yield false-negative results.[3] Such agents are β-adrenergic blocking drugs and centrally acting antisympathetic agents. Treatment with agents known to stimulate renin release are helpful in accentuating a significant renal venous renin differential. These include diuretics, ACE inhibitors, and angiotensin II-receptor antagonists and vasodilator agents. In addition, the renal venous blood samples should be obtained after several minutes of tilting the patient to further stimulate the renin system.[3] In general, a ratio of 1.5:1 or greater of the involved:uninvolved renal venous renin content (or the more-involved:less-involved, in the case of bilateral disease) is predictive of a functionally significant lesion and portends a favorable response to intervention.[3] In addition, in the case of unilateral renal vascular lesions, the contralateral renal venous concentration of renin should be equal to or lower than the levels in blood from the inferior vena cava remote from the drainage of the renal veins. This confirms that the involved kidney is the sole source of increased renin production. For a variety of reasons, *periph-*

eral venous renin content may be within the normal range and thus cannot be used as a reliable screening test.[3]

A variety of treatment options are available for patients with renal vascular hypertension. The current spectrum of antihypertensive agents, including drugs that interfere specifically with the renin-angiotensin system such as ACE inhibitors and the new angiotensin II-receptor blockers, can often control blood pressure in most patients with renal vascular disease. However, blood pressure control alone does not ensure improvement of either the obstructive lesion of the renal artery or the hemodynamic abnormality that it produces. Indeed, several studies have now demonstrated progression of renal impairment despite adequate blood pressure control with antihypertensive drug therapy.[6] Thus, improvement of the hemodynamic abnormality with restoration of renal perfusion is an important goal along with blood pressure reduction.

The two basic options to consider are surgery and percutaneous transluminal angioplasty. Surgical intervention typically involves endarterectomy and reanastomosis, a bypass graft procedure, or nephrectomy when the kidney cannot be salvaged. During the past 20 years, angioplasty, including the placement of stents for difficult lesions, has become an alternative to surgery. The experience with angioplasty is extensive and usually effective, even with severe atherosclerotic lesions. However, many patients also have evidence of diffuse atherosclerotic disease of the coronary and cerebral vessels, and thus are not always ideal surgical candidates. Moreover, when extensive fibrodysplasia of the renal arteries is encountered, typically in young women of premenopausal age, the disease may extend into the branching renal vessels, and thus is not always surgically correctible. In such cases, angioplasty has been effective.

The question often arises whether angioplasty should be the treatment of choice for all patients with renal vascular hypertension, irrespective of the etiology of the disease.

When the etiology of renal vascular hypertension is atherosclerotic, the lesions often extend into the aortic ostium of the renal artery, making it technically difficult to achieve effective dilatation. Cholesterol emboli to the kidney or distal aorta are common. Recurrence of the atheroma and subsequent restenosis are also common in the renal artery as they are in the coronary arteries after angioplasty. The procedure should be coupled with lipid-lowering strategies, smoking cessation, and antiplatelet aggregation (eg, aspirin) therapy to reduce the probability of recurrence. At the least, a program of careful, periodic evaluation of both blood pressure and renal function is required for the length of the patient's life.

Primary Aldosteronism

Primary aldosteronism is caused by the excessive production of aldosterone or other mineralocorticoids. The increased steroid production then promotes reabsorption of sodium and water and expansion of extracellular fluid volume with a resultant increase in blood pressure. The steroid-induced sodium reabsorption occurs through the exchange of sodium for potassium and hydrogen ions by the distal portion of the nephron, which typically produces hypokalemia and a metabolic alkalosis. When the kidneys are normal, the increase in volume, sodium content, and blood pressure serves to suppress renin, the usual primary stimulus for aldosterone production. Thus, the hallmark of mineralocorticoid-mediated hypertension is marked suppression of plasma renin levels.[7] Traditionally, serum potassium measurements are used to screen for primary aldosteronism. However, evidence indicates that as many as 25% of patients with primary aldosteronism may have serum potassium levels within the normal range (plasma potassium levels are generally lower than those for serum because of less hemolysis of erythrocytes).[8,9] Moreover, most patients with hypertension and hypokalemia have *secondary* aldosteronism from diuretic administration, renal vascular hypertension, etc. Therefore, serum potassium measurement alone is not a specific screening test for primary aldosteronism. When hypokalemia is present, some physicians advocate obtaining a 24-hour urinary potassium measurement to identify excessive potassium excretion. If this is done, measuring plasma renin activity is still necessary to differentiate between primary and secondary aldosteronism because renin is low in the former and high in the latter.

It is more cost efficient, therefore, to begin the screen for primary aldosteronism with the plasma renin measurement. However, a suppressed value is not diagnostic of primary aldosteronism because approximately 25% of those with essential hypertension (the low-renin subgroup) have suppressed renin levels. In addition, renin can be lowered by a high dietary salt intake, by a variety of antihypertensive drugs (eg, β-adrenergic blockers, antisympathetic agents), and by steroids.

The most specific screening test for primary aldosteronism is measuring plasma renin and plasma aldosterone in a single peripheral blood sample obtained while the patient is ambulatory (which stimulates renin levels).[10] A ratio of aldosterone to renin in excess of 30 (ng/dL:ng/mL/90 minutes) is diagnostic of primary aldosteronism (as long as the aldosterone values are >15). A ratio of 15 to 30 should raise strong suspicions of primary aldosteronism, particularly as related to bilateral adrenal disease (see discussion of subtypes below).

Another advantage of using the ratio as a screening test is that it can often be used even while the patient is receiving antihypertensive drugs, *as long as the impact of the specific agents on the renin-aldosterone system is considered.* For example, ACE inhibitors should increase renin and reduce aldosterone values. Thus, the observation of an abnormal ratio during ACE inhibitor treatment cannot be caused by the drug. As previously mentioned, β-blockers and antisympathetic drugs decrease renin, while calcium channel entry blockers increase renin and may reduce aldosterone slightly. Other antihypertensive agents, such as diuretics and vasodilators, increase renin levels. Thus, it is not always necessary to discontinue all antihypertensives to pursue an initial screen for primary aldosteronism. Renin measurements are indexed to urinary sodium excretion, or obtained after some stimulatory maneuver such as a low-salt diet or diuretic administration, and are often used as an initial screening test. If the test results are abnormal, a second measurement of the aldosterone level in plasma or urine is required to separate 'low-renin' essential hypertension from adrenal disease. This typically requires either a high-salt diet or an intravenous saline load to demonstrate inappropriate aldosterone production.[11] The cost, time, and relative insensitivity of such a sequential screening process is no longer justifiable in view of the efficiency, sensitivity, and specificity of the renin:aldosterone ratio.[10]

Once a diagnosis of primary aldosteronism is made, the etiology and location of the lesion must be determined to provide the most appropriate therapy. The classic form of primary aldosteronism, encountered in approximately 60% of such patients, is caused by a solitary (benign) adrenal adenoma.[8] These are usually small (less than 1 cm in diameter) and not easily identified by anatomic techniques such as computed tomography (CT) scanning or venography. In some recent studies, magnetic resonance imaging (MRI) and photon emission tomography (PET) scanning were used to identify unilateral adenomas. Approximately 30% of patients with primary aldosteronism have bilateral adrenal hyperproduction with both macronodules and micronodules.[8] Moreover, in this form of primary aldosteronism even bilateral adrenalectomy, which removes the increased steroid production, does not usually lead to lower blood pressure, and the patient is doomed to lifelong steroid replacement therapy. In contrast, when an unilateral adenoma is identified and removed, the hypertension as well as the hyperaldosteronism and its metabolic sequelae are usually cured. The remaining 10% of patients with primary aldosteronism consists of patients with bilateral solitary adenomas, adrenal carcinoma, unilateral macronodular and micronodular disease, and genetically mediated steroid biosynthetic abnormalities. Obviously, the treatment is different for these various forms, and differentiation is required after the diagnosis of primary aldosteronism is reached.

In general, two positive, confirmatory localizing tests are required before recommending surgical intervention for unilateral hyperaldosteronism.[8] A positive CT (or MRI or PET) scan is useful only if confirmed by another test. One such test is the anomalous postural decline in plasma aldosterone when comparing blood samples obtained at 8 AM after bedrest with those obtained at noon after 4 hours of ambulation. Typically, plasma levels of aldosterone should rise during this period. In many patients with unilateral adrenal disease, an anomalous fall is seen.[8] An adrenal radioisotopic scan can also be used to confirm unilateral disease. The most accurate localizing technique is an adrenal vein catheterization to sample venous blood for adrenal steroid concentration.[8] However, this must be done under very specific conditions, and the success of adrenal venous blood sampling depends on the skill and experience of the radiologist doing the procedure.

One approach is to sample from both adrenal veins and from the inferior vena cava at a site remote from adrenal venous drainage. Measurements of both aldosterone and cortisol concentration should be made and the latter used both to assess the purity of the adrenal vein blood sample and to correct for dilution of adrenal venous blood by nonadrenal effluent. Intravenous administration of adrenocorticotrophic hormone (ACTH) 30 minutes before and during the procedure can be used to maximize steroid production and to reduce error caused by episodic release of endogenous ACTH.[8] Then, the ratio of aldosterone to cortisol (disregarding the units of measurement) in blood from the adrenal veins is compared with that in the inferior vena cava. Finding aldosterone-to-cortisol ratios similar in blood from both adrenal veins and higher than that in the vena cava implies bilateral adrenal disease. An elevated ratio from one adrenal sample with the ratio from the contralateral gland similar to or lower than that in the inferior vena cava indicates unilateral aldosteronism.

Occasionally, blood cannot be obtained from one adrenal vein. In such instances, if the ratio from the sampled adrenal vein is lower than that in the inferior vena cava, it can be inferred that the unsampled adrenal vein is the source of increased aldosterone production. For adrenal vein blood to be adequate, the cortisol concentration (during ACTH stimulation) should be greater than 250 µg/dL. In the inferior vena cava sample, cortisol values of 25 to 50 µg/dL are anticipated. Curiously, the absolute values of aldosterone in the various blood samples are not diagnostic by themselves. A major ancillary benefit of identifying the site of a unilateral adrenal lesion is the option to choose the less morbid flank approach for adrenalectomy, as opposed to an abdominal incision with exploration of both adrenal glands. This is particularly valuable in view of the small size of most adrenal adenomas that cause primary aldosteronism. There are now several reports of laparoscopic adrenalectomy for this disorder.

In adrenal carcinoma, elevated values of other steroids, particularly urinary 17-ketosteroids, are observed. In addition, other manifestations of malignant disease may be seen. The identification of bilateral adrenal adenomas is difficult. Anatomic studies can be suggestive, but this rare situation is usually considered when a transient improvement of the syndrome of primary aldosteronism occurs after unilateral adrenalectomy, followed by a recurrence of the metabolic and hemodynamic alterations. Only recently has the mechanism been elucidated for the genetic disorders that may rarely cause primary aldosteronism.

A familial form of primary aldosteronism has been recognized for 30 years, but the manifestations are varied.[12] One form is responsive to long-term glucocorticoid administration, the dexamethasone-suppressible (DSH) or GRA variant.[12] Recently, it has been determined that this is the result of a chimerism of the 11β-hydroxylase and aldosterone synthase genes that leads to an ACTH-sensitive, aldosterone-producing adrenal zona glomerulosa.[13] Such individuals also produce increased levels of 18-hydroxycortisol and 18-oxocortisol in the urine. Again, because this abnormality involves both adrenal glands, total adrenalectomy is not usually desirable. These patients can be treated with glucocorticoid (dexamethasone in doses of 0.5 to 2.0 mg/d) or with potassium-sparing diuretic combinations that include thiazide diuretics with amiloride (Moduretic®), triamterene (Dyazide®), or spironolactone (Aldactazide®). In addition to potassium-sparing diuretic combinations, calcium channel entry blockers such as nifedipine (Procardia XL®) and verapamil (Calan® SR, Isoptin®) are also effective in some patients with primary aldosteronism caused by bilateral disease, both the genetic variant and the more common bilateral adrenal hyperplasia. In a small number of patients with bilateral adrenal involvement, aldosterone production appears to be exquisitely sensitive to angiotensin II. For this reason, ACE inhibitors and, theoretically, the ARBs may be effective in reducing aldosterone production and blood pressure. Regardless of the therapeutic choice, long-term follow-up is required for patients with primary aldosteronism.

Pheochromocytoma

Pheochromocytoma is an abnormality of the adrenal medulla or other sympathetic nervous system tissue that produces excess amounts of catecholamines. Because of its dramatic manifestations and because it tends to be severe and difficult to control, it is a particularly dangerous form of hypertension. Paroxysms of catecholamine release can precipitate not only marked fluctuations in blood pressure, but also sudden symptoms of congestive heart failure, acute myocardial infarction, or stroke. Contrary to popular belief, episodic hypertension is *not* a common finding in patients with pheochromocytoma, observed only in approximately 15% of cases, whereas the overwhelming majority of patients have sustained elevation of blood pressure.[2] However, marked increases in blood pressure can occur in association with any of a large number of activities that stimulate the sympathetic nervous system, such as defecation, sneezing, coughing, sexual intercourse, micturition, exercise, postural changes, abdominal palpation, smoking, or the ingestion of tyramine-rich foods such as red wine or hard cheeses.[2] Flushing of the skin is *not* typical in pheochromocytoma. In contrast, pallor and cold extremities are more typical because of intense cutaneous vasoconstriction. Sweating and severe headaches may occur. Palpitations and tachycardia, reflecting the effect of increased catecholamines on the heart, are also common. Tremulousness and a variety of other nonspecific symptoms have been reported in fewer than half of the patients with pheochromocytoma.

More common physical findings are hypertension, pallor, and severe retinopathy (grades III and IV) in more than half of patients with pheochromocytoma.[2] These findings are all related to the vasoconstrictor effects of increased catecholamines. Orthostatic hypotension may occur in some patients in whom epinephrine or dopamine production predominates. The diagnosis of pheochromocytoma should be considered when a patient has severe or refractory hypertension, when grades III or IV eyegrounds are present, when symptoms suggest the diagnosis, or when a hypertensive patient has other findings associated with this abnormality. These include cutaneous neurofibromas, cafe-au-lait skin lesions, gallstones, renal artery stenosis, and multiple endocrine neoplasia (MEN) syndromes.

The diagnosis of pheochromocytoma is complicated by the need for complete 24-hour urine collection and measurement of a variety of catecholamines and their metabolites (eg, vanillylmandelic acid, homovanillic acid, metanephrines) because of individual variability in the production and metabolism of catecholamines. Some investigators have advocated measurement of plasma catecholamines before and after administration of clonidine (Catapres®), an antihypertensive agent that normally acts to suppress sympathetic nervous system release of catecholamines. However, this approach often yields false-negative and false-positive results. One of the most specific screening tests for pheochromocytoma is the 'sleep' urinary norepinephrine measurement.[14] This reduces error induced by incomplete collection of a 24-hour urine sample or, in the unusual case of an episodically secreting tumor, dilution of the 24-hour catecholamine value by a long quiescent period. In addition, the sleep period represents a period of normal suppression of the sympathetic nervous system, which thereby enables easier recognition of even a mild increase in catecholamines as is virtually always present in pheochromocytoma, even when quiescent. The patient is asked to void and discard the urine before retiring and to note the time. All urine voided during the sleep period and directly after rising is collected; the duration of the sleep period is noted; and the sample is assayed for norepinephrine. In our experience, the highest value for patients with normal or essential hypertension is less than 35 µg/8 hours, whereas the *lowest* value for any patient with pheochromocytoma is more than 75 µg/8 hours, and usually more than 200 µg/8 hours.[14]

Most pheochromocytomas are located in the adrenal medulla, and approximately 90% are below the diaphragm.[2] These tumors are typically larger than 3 cm in diameter and, unlike adrenal adenomas that cause primary aldosteronism, are much easier to identify with noninvasive tests. There has been great success with CT scanning[15]; others have used MRI effectively. Sometimes, a plain x-ray of the abdomen shows a calcified mass in the adrenal area that represents hemorrhagic necrosis of parts of the tumor. Invasive procedures such as arteriography are rarely necessary to identify the site of the tumor. Such approaches may trigger a paroxysmal release of catecholamines and increase the risk of a vascular event. Occasionally, it is necessary to use radioisotopic scanning with metaiodobenzylguanidine to locate the tumor, particularly when multiple or metastatic lesions are suspected.

The surgical approach to pheochromocytoma requires special consideration. The process of dissecting to the tumor and isolating it can cause massive release of catecholamines and precipitate a vascular event, arrhythmia, or death. Although pharmacologic blockade of α-adrenergic and β-adrenergic receptors can be easily accomplished with intravenous administration during the surgery, this does not necessarily prevent the catastrophic event of profound refractory hypotension after tumor removal. This results from the intense vasoconstriction associated with the increased levels of catecholamines that serve to reduce extracellular fluid volume before surgery by reducing the vascular cross-sectional area and capacitance. When the source of increased catecholamines is suddenly removed during surgery, dramatic vasodilatation occurs in the presence of an underfilled vascular space. Sometimes, it is not possible to administer fluid rapidly enough to prevent profound hypotension and shock. Therefore, it is preferable to administer effective α-adrenergic blocking drugs and to titrate the dose to the presence of orthostatic hypotension for 7 to 10 days before surgery to permit the expansion of extracellular fluid volume before removal of the tumor. A familial incidence of pheochromocytoma requires screening of relatives for this problem. Long-term follow-up is also required for the involved patient because multiple or malignant tumors are not uncommon. When surgery is not an option or when metastatic disease is present, treatment with methylparatyrosine (Demser®) and/or α-adrenergic blocking agents such as phenoxybenzamine (Dibenzyline®), prazosin (Minipress®), terazosin (Hytrin®), or doxazosin (Cardura®) can be used.

Cushing's Syndrome

The best screening test for Cushing's syndrome is measurement of free cortisol in a 24-hour urine collection. Verification of the completeness of the urine collection can be accomplished by measuring creatinine excretion in the sample. Occasionally, the free cortisol value may be elevated in obese patients without Cushing's syndrome, but this is less likely than if 17β-hydroxysteroids are measured. In such instances, a dexamethasone suppression test (0.5 mg q 6 hours for 2 days) with the collection of a 24-hour urine sample during the second day should demonstrate marked suppression of urinary steroids in obese patients.

When the free cortisol value in the urine is elevated, studies to differentiate adrenal from pituitary causes are necessary. A variety of techniques are used for this purpose, but direct measurement of ACTH in plasma should permit separation of the forms. Pituitary Cushing's syndrome is associated with elevated ACTH levels and should be followed by CT or MRI scan of the pituitary to identify a lesion. Occasionally, ectopic ACTH production by a malignant tumor may be present, but such patients typically have other manifestations of malignant disease. When ACTH levels are suppressed, the etiology is likely to be adrenal. Computed tomography scans may identify an adrenal tumor.

Thyroid Disorders

Hypertension may occur with hypothyroidism or hyperthyroidism. With the latter, systolic hypertension and tachycardia are common and reflect the increased sympathetic drive associated with elevated thyroid hormone levels. In hypothyroidism, elevation of diastolic pressure is more common and bradycardia is often present. Typically, patients with thyroid disease and hypertension also have other signs or symptoms of the underlying thyroid disorder. In the elderly, however, the manifestations of thyroid disease may be obscured by the reduced sympathetic responsiveness. The diagnosis of either form of thyroid disease can usually be established by measurement of plasma thyroxine (or triiodothyronine) and thyroid-stimulating hormone (TSH) levels. In hyperthyroidism, the circulating thyroid hormone levels are elevated, and TSH may be increased to suggest a pituitary etiology or decreased to suggest primary thyroid overactivity. In hypothyroidism, circulating thyroid hormone levels are low and TSH is typically increased to stimulate more thyroid hormone secretion. A variety of treatment options are available, depending on the etiology of the disease. In hypothyroidism, thyroid replacement therapy requires frequent calibration because a variety of circumstances may alter the bioeffectiveness of therapy. This is particularly important for patients with hypertension who receive thyroid replacement therapy because increased or decreased 'effective' thyroid hormone levels may modify blood pressure and the ability to control it with antihypertensive agents. Thyroxine and TSH levels should be checked annually in patients who receive thyroid replacement therapy.

Collagen Vascular Disease

When hypertension is related to a collagen vascular disorder (eg, systemic lupus erythematosus, scleroderma, periarteritis nodosa, etc), it usually reflects renal involvement with the vasculitic process. Thus, evidence of impaired renal function, based both on elevated BUN or creatinine values and on reduced creatinine clearance or the presence of erythrocytes or protein in the urine, usually suggests the underlying problem. Appropriate diagnosis and treatment is obvious. Because the hypertension is usually of renal etiology, it is often associated with increased renin release, in effect producing a 'high-renin' form of hypertension. Not surprisingly, ACE inhibitors have been effective in many of these patients not only in achieving blood pressure control, but also in decreasing the extent of renal damage.

Perinephritis

The 'Page' kidney results from hemorrhage-induced perinephritis, and usually results from trauma. Often, the injury is long forgotten when the elevated blood pressure is discovered. Mild renal impairment may be present. When hypertension is noted in a young individual, particularly one involved in athletics or in someone without a family history of hypertension, an evaluation of renal function should be performed. Anatomic and functional tests are necessary. The 'Page' kidney has been classically identified with intravenous pyelography or arteriography. Isotopic renal scans should be able to detect the reduced blood flow and structural distortion of the renal profile in this disorder, but no reports have appeared in the literature to confirm this. Treatment generally requires surgical decompression of the kidney or, in some cases, nephrectomy.

Brachydactyly-Hypertension Syndrome

It has recently been observed in a rural clan of Turkish shepherds and their families that severe hypertension with its vascular sequelae and shortened lifespan exist in concert with short fingers, but not with other obvious skeletal or endocrine abnormalities.[16] In family members without short fingers, blood pressure and lifespan are completely normal. Additional studies may elucidate the genetic mediation of this abnormality and the mechanism(s) by which it occurs.

References

1.   Scott PL, Yune HY, Weinberger MH: Page kidney: an unusual cause of hypertension. *Radiology* 1976;119:547-548.

2.   Manger WM, Gifford RW Jr: *Pheochromocytoma*. Springer-Verlag, New York, 1977, pp 85-135.

3.   Grim CE, Luft FC, Weinberger MH, et al: Sensitivity and specificity of screening tests for renal vascular hypertension. *Ann Intern Med* 1979;91:617-622.

4.   Fommei E, Ghione S, Palla L, et al: Renal scintigraphic captopril test in the diagnosis of renovascular hypertension. *Hypertension* 1987;10:212-220.

5.   Zabbo A, Novick AC: Digital subtraction angiography for noninvasive imaging of the renal artery. *Urol Clin North Am* 1984;11:409-416.

6. Hunt JC, Sheps SG, Harrison EG, et al: Renal and renovascular hypertension: a reasoned approach to diagnosis and management. *Arch Intern Med* 1974;988:133-137.

7. Conn JW, Cohen EL, Rovner DR: Suppression of plasma renin activity in primary aldosteronism. *JAMA* 1964;190:213-221.

8. Weinberger MH, Grim CE, Hollifield JW, et al: Primary aldosteronism: diagnosis, localization and treatment. *Ann Intern Med* 1979;90:386-395.

9. Gordon RD, Klemm SA, Tunny TJ, et al: Primary aldosteronism: hypertension with a genetic basis. *Lancet* 1992;340:159-161.

10. Weinberger MH, Fineberg NS: The diagnosis of primary aldosteronism and separation of two major subtypes. *Arch Intern Med* 1993;153:2125-2129.

11. Kem DC, Weinberger MH, Mayes DM, et al: Saline suppression of plasma aldosterone in hypertension. *Arch Intern Med* 1971; 128:380-386.

12. Sutherland DJ, Ruse JL, Laidlaw JC: Hypertension, increased aldosterone secretion and low plasma renin activity relieved by dexamethasone. *Can Med Assoc J* 1966;95:1109-1119.

13. Lifton RP, Dluhy RG, Powers M, et al: A chimaeric 11β-hydroxylase/aldosterone synthase gene causes glucocorticoid-remediable aldosteronsim and human hypertension. *Nature* 1992; 355:262-265.

14. Ganguly A, Henry DP, Yune HY, et al: Diagnosis and localization of pheochromocytoma: detection by measurement of urinary norepinephrine during sleep, plasma norepinephrine concentration and computed axial tomography (CT-scan). *Am J Med* 1979;67:21-26.

15. Ganguly A, Pratt JH, Yune HY, et al: Detection of adrenal tumors by computerized tomographic scan in endocrine hypertension. *Arch Intern Med* 1979;139:589-592.

16. Schuster H, Wienker TF, Bahring S, et al: Severe autosomal dominant hypertension and brachydactyly in a unique Turkish kindred maps to human chromosome 12. *Nat Genet* 1996;13:98-100.

Chapter 5

Nonpharmacologic Treatment and Primary Prevention

Numerous lifestyle factors are associated with elevated blood pressure (Table 5-1). Identification of these factors and of individual susceptibilities regarding blood pressure may often allow for specific nonpharmacologic approaches to treatment and prevention of hypertension. The importance of the latter has been reflected by the change in nomenclature of the main committee establishing guidelines for hypertension, the Joint National Committee on Prevention, Detection, Evaluation, and Treatment of High Blood Pressure.[1]

Obesity

Obesity has long been associated with elevated blood pressure. A recent study demonstrated that upper body (abdominal) obesity (the android or 'apple' shape) is associated with elevated blood pressure, insulin resistance, dyslipidemia, and increased cardiovascular disease risk. The predominantly lower body pattern of obesity is referred to as the gynecoid or 'pear' shape.[2] An overabundance of mesenteric fat has also been identified as a major component in the relationship between obesity and blood pressure. Although the association is well recognized, the mechanisms involved are not clear.

One partial explanation for the relationship between obesity and blood pressure may be related to the blood

Table 5-1: Lifestyle Factors Influencing Blood Pressure

- nutrition
- obesity
- sodium
- potassium
- calcium
- caffeine
- omega-3 fish oils
- vitamin C
- excessive alcohol consumption
- lack of exercise
- stress

pressure measurement itself. As mentioned in Chapter 1, the indirect method requires the use of a cuff that is sized appropriately for the circumference of the patient's arm. Thus, the blood pressure reading of an obese patient may be artificially elevated if it is taken with an average-sized cuff. In addition, not all obese patients have elevated blood pressure even when the proper cuff is used. Notwithstanding these findings, many patients with hypertension are obese, and, in some, weight loss of as little as 10 pounds may be associated with a significant reduction in blood pressure.[3] Thus, it is not always necessary for body weight to be reduced to the 'ideal' to yield a beneficial effect on blood pressure. It is important to recognize that not all obese patients with hypertension can lower their blood pressure by losing weight, and that maintaining weight loss requires lifestyle changes and long-term commitment. Finally, the pharmacologic agents traditionally used to enhance weight loss and dieting, such as amphetamines and phenylpropanolamine, can themselves raise blood pressure.

Sodium Intake

Sodium (salt) intake has long been linked to blood pressure.[4] Extensive literature, ranging from epidemiologic to interventional studies, confirms the finding that elevated blood pressure and its cardiovascular consequences are rare among societies in which habitual sodium intake is lower than 50 to 100 mmoL (mEq) per day. These observations are confounded by many other components, such as calcium and potassium intake, exercise, and cultural and genetic differences.[4] In addition, skeptics of the salt-blood pressure hypothesis have pointed out that not all individuals demonstrate changes in blood pressure when sodium intake is altered, and conclude that salt is not an important factor in the pathogenesis or treatment of hypertension. The most dramatic reductions in blood pressure were observed with severe salt restriction to levels of less than 1 g/d. Because such levels are difficult for many patients to maintain without the purchase of special foods, some clinicians have concluded that salt restriction is impractical except under investigational circumstances or in institutional environments. However, it has been consistently shown that even modest reduction of salt intake to levels of 2 to 3 g/d can lower blood pressure in many patients with hypertension, and can be maintained without undue expense or difficulty.[5] Such reduction in salt intake requires some understanding of the sources of salt in processed and prepared foods, and a willingness to read food labels.

A greater insight into the role of salt in human blood pressure came from the repeated demonstration of the heterogeneity of responses in both healthy and hypertensive patients.[4] It is now clear that some individuals have blood pressure levels that are sensitive to alterations in dietary sodium and extracellular fluid volume, whereas others do not. Evidence indicates that 50% to 60% of the hypertensive population, and about 25% of the normotensives are salt sensitive.[6] Salt sensitivity of blood pressure is more common among black hypertensives than in white patients, and increases with age in both healthy and hypertensive groups.[6] This appears to contribute to the increase both in blood pressure and in the prevalence of hypertension with increasing age.[7] Although there are no simple tests to identify salt sensitivity of blood pressure, a decrease in blood pressure after 7 to 10 days of diuretic therapy strongly suggests the possibility that patients with hypertension who have no identifiable response to diuretics are likely to be salt resistant.

Modest salt restriction lowered blood pressure to the normal range in some patients with hypertension, which eliminated the need for drug treatment.[5] Moreover, even in drug-treated hypertension, salt restriction enhances blood pressure control and frequently reduces the need for antihypertensive medication.[5] Measurement of 24-hour urinary sodium excretion is the best indicator of sodium intake, and can be used to determine whether a patient is successful or compliant with prescribed dietary regimens.

Potassium Intake

Potassium is a factor in blood pressure levels. Although its role is less impressive than sodium, both epidemiologic and interventional observations support the importance of this nutrient. Potassium intake is often inversely related to that of sodium, so that high-sodium diets are typically associated with low potassium intake, and vice versa. However, the observations about the effect of potassium supplementation on blood pressure are inconsistent. In studies of hypertensives, potassium supplementation appears to have the greatest effect in lowering blood pressure among those who are potassium-depleted because they are taking a diuretic or because they have a diet deficient in potassium.[8] This heterogeneity in response to potassium may account for the relatively weak effect of this ion in studies of mixed hypertensive populations. Independent of the blood pressure effects of potassium, this nutrient is shown to have a powerful vascular-protective effect, particularly against stroke.[9] A dietary intake of potassium-rich foods (fresh vegetables, fresh fruit, etc) of at least 60 to 80 mEq/d is recommended to avoid potassium depletion in untreated individuals. Patients with renal impairment should not receive potassium supplementation because of the risk of hyperkalemia. A recent study[10] indicates that a diet moderately reduced in sodium content, and high in fruits, vegetables, and low-fat dairy products can lower blood pressure in hypertensives.

Calcium

The role of calcium in blood pressure control is controversial and vigorously debated.[11,12] Epidemiologic support for decreased dietary calcium intake for hypertension has been suggested, but some studies have reported contradictory evidence.[13] Similarly, the results of interventional studies are inconsistent and modest at best. Again, these apparently inconsistent findings can be explained on the basis of heterogeneity of blood pressure responsiveness. Indeed, in one study conducted by our group, using a placebo-controlled, double-blind, randomized trial in both healthy and hypertensive subjects, we found no significant effect of calcium supplementation on blood pressure in the entire group.[14] However, when the population was separated for salt sensitivity of blood pressure, which was established earlier in the same subjects, marked differences in responses were seen. In those who were salt sensitive, calcium supplementation resulted in a significant fall in blood pressure in both healthy and hypertensive individuals. In the salt-resistant group, calcium supplementation was associated with an increase in blood pressure. When the entire group was considered, without respect to prior salt responsiveness of blood pressure, no significant effect of calcium was observed.[14] Based on these and other observations, it is recommended that adults consume at least 1,000 mg/d of calcium in diet or as a supplement.

Caffeine

A small number of studies have been performed to examine the effect of caffeine on blood pressure. However, a rigorous study design was not always used and, therefore, the results may not be definitive.[1] The best studies used decaffeinated and caffeinated beverages given in a blinded and randomized fashion to coffee-naive subjects. Under such conditions, small increases in blood pressure occurred with caffeine administration. In other trials that involved habitual coffee drinkers, no such effect was observed. Thus, it is possible that the effect of caffeine on blood pressure may only be observed in those who do not habitually drink coffee.

Omega-3 Fish Oils

A limited number of studies examined the role of omega-3 fish oils on blood pressure. By and large, these studies did not provide an antihypertensive role for fish oils in reasonable amounts.[1] Nevertheless, there is substantial evidence for a beneficial effect of omega-3 fish oils in reducing the risk of cardiovascular disease.

Vitamin C

Several studies suggested a possible blood pressure-lowering effect of vitamin C (ascorbic acid), but the required doses are not clear. In both epidemiologic and interventional studies, vitamin C has been consistently shown to reduce vascular events, presumably by its antioxidant effects.

Alcohol

A biphasic relationship between alcohol and blood pressure has been observed. Small amounts of alcohol are associated with vasodilatation and a slight fall in blood pressure. As alcohol consumption increases, blood pressure rises, presumably because of the effect on sympathetic nervous system activity and cardiac output. Habitual consumption of more than 1 oz of pure alcohol per day (representing 2 oz of 100-proof spirits, 8 oz of wine, or 24 oz of beer) is often associated with elevated blood pressure. Reduction in alcohol intake in such individuals usually lowers blood pressure and, in some cases, may be all that is required to achieve normal blood pressure levels.[13] Asking the patient about his or her alcohol consumption is an important part of the history, and may suggest a simple approach to treatment of hypertension.

Exercise

Sedentary lifestyle is associated with obesity, elevated blood pressure, and an increased risk for cardiovascular disease. Regular exercise is useful in maintaining ideal body weight, or weight loss in the obese, and also increases cardiovascular fitness. Few studies have examined the effects of exercise on blood pressure with controls for the confounding effect of weight loss that typically occurs when sedentary individuals begin a regular exercise program. Depending on the type, intensity, and duration of exercise, blood pressure may increase, stay the same, or decrease during exercise. For example, weightlifting is associated with marked elevation of blood pressure, with some of the highest measurements ever recorded in normal subjects. Other forms of vigorous exercise such as running, stair-stepping, and vigorous bicycling are also known to raise blood pressure. During the 'cooling off' period, assuming substantial effort expenditure, vasodilatation and fluid loss from perspiration are usually associated with a reduction in blood pressure below basal values. When the presence of vascular disease does not preclude regular exercise, effort should be made to pursue a gradual program of exercise progressing to 30 minutes or more at least 5 days per week of whatever activity is best suited for the individual. This may range from brisk walking to rapid running, stair-stepping, cycling, or engaging in vigorous sports. This degree of activity is shown to have beneficial cardiovascular effects and to raise HDL levels. The key is to select a program that the patient enjoys and is likely to maintain, and to begin the program gradually, building up to effective levels over weeks or months.

Stress

A relationship between stress and blood pressure has long been assumed, not only among the lay public but also among physicians. However, critical scientific demonstration of this relationship has been elusive for several reasons. First, there are no generally acceptable definitions or measures of stress. The responses to a variety of external and internal stimuli vary for each individual, and what one person perceives as stressful may not be so for someone else. In addition, it is difficult to identify a mechanism by which such an effect may be mediated. The sympathetic nervous system is often suggested as the operant mediator of stressful responses, but even this is difficult to measure accurately. Finally, there is no evidence that routinely used tranquilizers in doses insufficient to cause sleep or coma have any consistent antihypertensive effect.

After building an argument against a relationship between stress and blood pressure, it is also necessary to examine some of the evidence in its support. Using both 24-hour ambulatory blood pressure recording devices that permit noninvasive sampling of pressure as often as every 15 minutes, and more invasive, constant-monitoring techniques, the resulting data unequivocally demonstrate that blood pressure is extremely variable, and that this variability is clearly associated with activity and stress. Even among healthy individuals, blood pressure increases with both physical and emotional activity and reaches a nadir during sleep. The same pattern typically occurs in patients with hypertension. In either group, nocturnal (sleeping) pressures may be half of those observed during the most active or stressful times of the day. However, stress alone cannot account for the persistent elevation of blood pressure above the normal range that characterizes hypertension. An abnormality of the vascular or cardiac response to stress must also be involved.

Although tranquilizers in doses that permit lucidity do not consistently lower blood pressure in hypertension, other interventions were shown to have an effect. Biofeedback, transcendental meditation, and other relaxation techniques do indeed lower blood pressure in healthy and in hypertensive subjects. However, the reduction in blood pressure is usually transient and does not generally persist once the activity is ended.[1] Thus, except in rare individuals, stress management has not been shown to be an effective way of treating hypertension, and no information is available about the effect of stress management on the sequelae of hypertension.

Primary Prevention of Hypertension

The tests used to identify individuals destined to develop hypertension are imprecise. This has hampered the evaluation of definitive prevention techniques. However, the rapid progress in the identification of genetic markers for several types of hypertension should soon make it possible to identify susceptible individuals for primary prevention approaches. Despite this imprecision in identification, there are some risk factors that a small number of studies have attempted to link to primary prevention. For example, individuals defined as having high-normal blood pressure (diastolic pressure 85 to 89 mm Hg) are more likely to develop fixed hypertension over time.[1] Recent studies in such a population showed that nonpharmacologic approaches can reduce the number of patients who develop fixed hypertension compared with a control group.[10]

A genetic basis is indicated in that hypertension occurs more often both in families with probands who are hypertensive and in each of a pair of identical twins more often than in fraternal twins. However, shared environmental or cultural factors could also be involved. Hypertension is more common in African Americans than in whites. Individuals of Asian descent, especially Japanese or Chinese, also appear to have a higher incidence of hypertension. The prevalence of hypertension increases with age, but only in societies in which sodium intake is high. Moreover, individuals who are salt sensitive are more likely to have an age-related increase in blood pressure than those who are not salt sensitive, even within the normotensive population.[7]

These findings can help identify high-risk subjects before the development of hypertension. Then, a program of weight control, regular exercise, modest reduction of salt intake, increased potassium and calcium intake, and moderation in alcohol consumption may prevent the subsequent development of hypertension.[1] Moreover, there are no known harmful effects involved in any of these modest lifestyle and nutritional habits.

References

1. The Joint National Committee on Prevention, Detection, Evaluation, and Treatment of High Blood Pressure (JNC VI): the sixth report. *Arch Intern Med* 1997;157:2413-2446.

2. Despraes JP, Moorjani S, Lupien PJ, et al: Regional distribution of body fat, plasma lipoproteins, and cardiovascular disease. *Arteriosclerosis* 1990;10:497-511.

3. Schotte DE, Stunkard AJ: The effects of weight reduction on blood pressure in 301 obese patients. *Arch Intern Med* 1990; 150:1701-1704.

4. Weinberger MH: Salt sensitivity of blood pressure in humans. *Hypertension* 1996;27:481-490.

5. Weinberger MH, Cohen SJ, Miller JZ, et al: Dietary sodium restriction as adjunctive treatment of hypertension. *JAMA* 1988; 259:2561-2565.

6. Weinberger MH, Miller JZ, Luft FC, et al: Definitions and characteristics of sodium sensitivity and blood pressure resistance. *Hypertension* 1986;8:127-134.

7. Weinberger MH, Fineberg NS: Sodium and volume sensitivity of blood pressure: age and blood pressure change over time. *Hypertension* 1991;18:67-71.

8. Tobian L: The protective effects of high-potassium diets in hypertension, and the mechanisms by which high NaCl diets produce hypertension. A personal view. In: Laragh JH, Brenner BM,

eds. *Hypertension: Pathophysiology, Diagnosis, and Management,* 2nd ed. New York, Raven Press, 1995, pp 299-312.

9.   Khaw KT, Barrett-Connor E: Dietary potassium and stroke-associated mortality: a 12-year prospective population study. *N Engl J Med* 1987;316:235-240.

10. Appel LF, Moore TJ, Obarzanek E, et al, for the DASH Collaborative Study Group: A clinical trial of the effects of dietary patterns on blood pressure. *N Engl J Med* 1997;336:1116-1124.

11. MacGregor GA: Sodium is more important than calcium in essential hypertension. *Hypertension* 1985;7:628-637.

12. McCarron DA: Is calcium more important than sodium in the pathogenesis of essential hypertension? *Hypertension* 1985; 7:607-627.

13. Harlan WR, Harlan LC: Blood pressure and calcium and magnesium intake. In: Laragh JH, Brenner BM, eds. *Hypertension: Pathophysiology, Diagnosis, and Management,* 2nd ed. New York, Raven Press, 1995, pp 1143-1154.

14. Weinberger MH, Wagner UL, Fineberg NS: The blood pressure effects of calcium supplementation in humans of known sodium responsiveness. *Am J Hypertens* 1993;6:799-805.

Chapter 6

Drug Therapy: Attacking Extracellular Fluid Volume Expansion—Diuretics and Natriuretic Agents

The development of antihypertensive drug therapy, as with the treatment of many other disorders, has progressed from an empiric basis to more specific approaches. One example is the use of diuretic therapy. As mentioned in Chapter 5, 50% to 60% of the hypertensive population is salt sensitive. In this condition, blood pressure responds to manipulation of sodium and extracellular fluid volume changes. This relatively recent finding provides an explanation for why diuretic therapy is traditionally one of the first considerations for the treatment of hypertension.

Introduced in 1957, chlorothiazide was one of the earliest drugs used to reduce blood pressure. It became the cornerstone of multiple-drug antihypertensive therapy because of its availability and relative efficacy based on the results of the Veteran's Administration Cooperative Study in hypertension. This study was conducted shortly after the introduction of chlorothiazide and provided the rationale for multiple-drug (triple or stepped-care) therapy in the treatment of hypertension.[1] Notably, the participants in the VA Cooperative Study were all older men, and included a substantial number of African Americans. Both of these demographic traits are associated with an increased likelihood of salt sensitivity of blood pressure. Thus, it is not surprising that the therapeutic formula chosen for the study was effective in lowering blood pressure in this group.

Moreover, the VA Cooperative Study was one of the first to demonstrate the benefit of blood pressure reduction in hypertension by showing a decreased incidence of cardiovascular morbidity and mortality among treated patients, compared with those who received a placebo. Indeed, because of the impressive differences in outcomes between the two groups, the study was terminated earlier than planned so that the placebo group could receive the benefits of treatment. For ethical reasons, these observations have made it difficult to conduct placebo-controlled studies in any patients but those with the mildest hypertension.

Mechanisms of Action

Many clinicians initially believed that the blood pressure reduction that occurs with diuretics was caused solely by their abilities to reduce extracellular fluid (plasma) volume. However, it has been difficult to demonstrate that there is an initial increase in plasma volume in patients with hypertension and that diuretic treatment produces a sustained reduction in plasma volume. The failure to demonstrate an expanded plasma volume in untreated hypertensives does not rule out a role for this factor in hypertension, because a reduced vascular capacity may also exist from the vasoconstriction and rarefaction of tertiary arterioles. Thus, the 'normal' plasma volume may be inappropriate for the reduced vascular system. Moreover, the initial effect of diuretic therapy appears to be to reduce plasma volume, which results in the immediate effect on blood pressure. However, there is also a slower component of diuretic-associated blood pressure reduction that might not be observed for weeks or months.[2] This is attributed to the effects of diuretics on the vascular wall that reduce the water content within and enhance vasodilation. Finally, it has been shown that di-

Table 6-1: Diuretics and Their Doses (mg/d)

Proximal-Tubule Agents
benzthiazide (Exna®) 25-100

chlorothiazide (Diuril®) 250-1000

chlorthalidone (Hygroton®, Thalitone) 25-100

hydrochlorothiazide (Esidrix®, HydroDIURIL®, Oretic®) 12.5-100

hydroflumethazide (Diucardin®) 25-200

indapamide (Lozol®) 1.25-5

methylclothiazide (Enduron®) 2.5-10

metolazone (Mykrox®) 0.5-1.0

metolazone (Zaroxlyn®) 2.5-5.0

Loop
bumetanide (Bumex®) 0.5-2.0

ethacrynic acid (Edecrin®) 25-100

furosemide (Lasix®) 40-240

torsemide (Demadex®) 5-10

Potassium-Sparing
amiloride (Midamor®) 5-10

spironolactone (Aldactone®) 25-100

triamterene (Dyrenium®) 25-75

Combination Thiazide and Potassium-Sparing
With amiloride (Moduretic®) 50+5

With spironolactone (Aldactazide®) 25+25

With triamterene (Dyazide®, Maxzide®) 25+37.5; 50+75

uretic-induced volume depletion alters vascular responsiveness to pressor substances such as angiotensin II and norepinephrine.

Drugs, Sites of Action, and Doses

Despite the large number of diuretics available, these agents can be separated into three groups (Table 6-1) based on sites of action: (1) proximal-tubule, thiazide-type; (2) loop; and (3) potassium-sparing agents. Within each group, the drugs can be classified based on duration of action, dose, and cost.

The prototype of the proximal-tubule agents is hydro-chlorothiazide (HydroDIURIL®, Esidrix®, Oretic®), although a host of other sulfonamide diuretics have similar actions and efficacy. Initial studies with the diuretic agents in hypertension used dosages of as much as 2,000 mg/d of chlorothiazide (Diuril®) and 100 mg/d or more of hydro-chlorothiazide. For both agents, the dose-response curve in hypertension was demonstrated to be flat at dosages above 500 mg/d and 50 mg/d, respectively. Because the adverse effects of diuretics are dose dependent and because the blood pressure-lowering effect does not require the large doses used initially, there has been a great reduction in the dosage of diuretic used in the treatment of uncomplicated hypertension.[3] Unfortunately, dosages of hydrochlorothi-azide (or its equivalent in other agents of this class) below 25 mg/d have not been effective in most patients when used alone to reduce blood pressure and, thus, 'low-dose' di-uretic therapy generally requires an addition of another an-tihypertensive agent. This issue is subsequently addressed in greater detail.

Another representative of the proximal-tubule diuretic group, chlorthalidone (Hygroton®), has been used in many investigative studies. Typical starting dosages of this agent are 25 mg/d. The duration of action of all the drugs in this group is sufficiently long (10 to 16 hours) to permit dosing once per day, except for chlorothiazide (Diuril®), which must be given twice daily for optimal efficacy. In patients with renal impairment, most of the thiazide diuretics, ex-cept for indapamide (Lozol®) and metolazone (Zaroxolyn®, Mykrox®), do not appear to be effective.

The adverse effects of this class of diuretics are largely related to the mechanism of action. As mentioned, these effects are dose dependent and are observed at dosages of more than 12.5 mg/d of hydrochlorothiazide or chlorthalidone, or equivalent doses of the other agents in the group.

The most consistent finding is potassium loss. This results from the diuretic effects on the proximal tubule and also from the activation of the renin-angiotensin-aldosterone system that accompanies the diuretic-induced reduction in extracellular fluid volume. The increased aldosterone levels, in turn, promote sodium reabsorption in the collecting portion of the kidneys in exchange for potassium and hydrogen ions, which are excreted in the urine. Thus, the magnitude of diuretic-related potassium loss depends on the degree of renin-aldosterone system stimulation *and* on the amount of sodium reaching the collecting system. Serum potassium levels invariably decrease when effective doses of diuretics are given to individuals with normal renal function, unless sodium restriction, potassium supplementation, or other agents are used to combat this loss. Moreover, serum potassium levels are relatively insensitive to the changes in intracellular potassium concentration, where more than 90% of the body's potassium stores are found. Alterations of intracellular potassium content appear to be responsible for the muscle cramps and arrhythmias associated with potassium loss. The latter may contribute to sudden death that appears to increase in hypertensive patients treated with diuretics.[4,5] Thiazide-induced magnesium loss may also contribute to these events. Thiazides can also cause hypercalcemia.

In addition to their effects on potassium and magnesium, thiazide diuretics obviously influence sodium balance. In most individuals, the compensatory effects of the renin-angiotensin-aldosterone system to maintain sodium balance and of the vasopressin system to maintain plasma osmolality in the normal range prevent the possible harm from diuretic-related sodium and water loss. In some individuals, typically elderly women, the compensatory systems do not function properly, and sudden, profound hyponatremia can occur with initial diuretic treatment. For this reason, it is important to obtain baseline electrolyte measurements, to begin with low doses of diuretic, and to monitor electrolyte and clinical status, particularly in high-risk individuals. In addition, in the rare instances when significant hyponatremia occurs, slow repletion of sodium stores is indicated to avoid rapid osmotic changes and the risk of cerebral and cerebellar demyelinization.

Electrolyte changes are not the only alterations that occur with thiazide diuretics. Hyperuricemia is common, and acute attacks of gout occasionally occur. Other alterations associated with thiazide treatment include hyperglycemia, which may precipitate or exacerbate diabetes mellitus resulting from insulin resistance and perhaps other effects of diuretic treatment.[6] Hyperlipidemia may also occur with diuretic therapy, and manifests primarily by elevations of total cholesterol and triglycerides.[7] Despite the statements of some investigators, these are not transient changes, but persist for the duration of treatment, based on offset observations in long-term diuretic treatment trials.[7]

A variety of other side effects occur with diuretics. Thiazide diuretics can also cause or worsen sexual dysfunction, a common problem in men with hypertension.[3] In addition to occasional nausea and constipation, thiazides can rarely cause pancreatitis or episodes of abdominal and back pain. In these circumstances, the drug should probably be stopped. Skin rash is another occasional side effect; rarely, hematologic changes such as thrombocytopenia, agranulocytosis, and anemia have been observed.

Loop Diuretics

These drugs work at the loop of Henle in the renal tubule, and are effective even when renal function is reduced, unlike most of the proximal-tubule thiazide agents. Furosemide (Lasix®) is the prototype of this class of drugs, which also includes bumetanide (Bumex®), ethacrynic acid (Edecrin®), and torsemide (Demadex®). Furosemide is a short-acting diuretic that lasts for 4 to 5 hours and, thus, must be given 3 to 4 times a day for optimal antihypertensive efficacy. Bumetanide and torsemide are sufficiently long acting to be effective once a day. Because all of these agents are potent, they are useful in edematous states, acute pulmonary edema, renal failure, and other situations in which rapid diuresis is required. However, they are not indicated for most patients with uncomplicated hypertension, for whom thiazide diuretics are preferable. All of the loop diuretics share the same dose-dependent adverse effects of the thiazide drugs, with the possible exception of hypercalcemia, which does not usually occur with loop agents.

Potassium-Sparing Agents

The agents acting at the distal nephron site to conserve potassium include spironolactone (Aldactone®), triamterene (Dyrenium®), and amiloride (Midamor®). The latter two agents have weak diuretic effects and are often combined with thiazide (Dyazide®, Maxzide®, and Moduretic®). In general, these agents should not be used in patients with renal failure or in diabetic patients with hyporeninemic hypoaldosteronism because of the risk of hyperkalemia. If a potassium-sparing agent is used in these populations, careful monitoring of renal function and potassium is required. Similarly, these drugs should be used cautiously in patients receiving potassium supplementation, angiotensin-converting enzyme (ACE) inhibitors, or angiotensin II receptor blockers because of the risk of hyperkalemia. The potassium-sparing agents alone do not demonstrate the adverse effects associated with the thiazide agents, but when the two are used in combination, some of these adverse effects may occur. The rationale for the use of potassium-sparing drugs is to blunt or prevent potassium loss, particularly that associated with other diuretics. Triamterene has a shorter half-life than the other two agents and must be given twice a day to counteract the effects of thiazide-induced potassium loss. The other combinations can be given effectively once a day.

Spironolactone may cause painful gynecomastia and impotence in men or mastodynia and menstrual irregularities in women. Triamterene may cause renal calculi. An adverse reaction has been reported between potassium-sparing drugs and nonsteroidal anti-inflammatory drugs (NSAIDs) with resultant hyperkalemia and renal impairment.

Combination Agents

The combination of thiazide and potassium-sparing agents was reviewed earlier. Concerns about the adverse effects of diuretics when used in the large doses required to achieve blood pressure control have resulted in a growing interest in the use of low-dose diuretics in combination with other nondiuretic antihypertensive agents. *Low-dose* refers to dosages of less than 25 mg/d of hydrochlorothiazide or chlorthalidone. For example, combinations of the β-adrenergic blocking agent bisoprolol with 6.25 mg of hydrochlorothiazide (Ziac®) have demonstrated greater efficacy than the β-blocker alone. This approach is particularly effective because many nondiuretic antihypertensive agents may develop decreased efficacy because of compensatory fluid retention and volume expansion. This is called *pseudotolerance*. Therefore, the combination of a low-dose diuretic with another nondiuretic antihypertensive agent provides improved efficacy and reduces the adverse effects of full-dose diuretic therapy.

Calcium Channel Entry Blockers

Although the drugs of the calcium channel blocking class are reviewed in greater detail in Chapter 7, their effects on extracellular fluid volume should be cited here in relation to their vasodilatory actions. A common side effect of many of the calcium channel entry blockers is dependent edema, which leads to the common misconception that these agents induce fluid retention and volume expansion. In fact, calcium channel blockers have been shown to have a natriuretic and diuretic effect similar to that of thiazide diuretics.[8] It appears that the dependent edema that often occurs with these agents is a reflection of capillary vasodilation and escape of fluid from the vascular to the interstitial space.[9] In general, edema associated with calcium channel blocker therapy is more responsive to postural alterations (periodic elevation of the feet), support stockings to reduce dependent edema, and, rarely, the use of small doses of ACE inhibitors that appear to act by reducing postcapillary pressure, than to diuretics.

References

1.   Veterans Administration Cooperative Study Group on Antihypertensive Agents: Effects of treatment on morbidity in hypertension: results in patients with diastolic blood pressure averaging 115 through 129 mm Hg. *JAMA* 1967;202:1028-1034.

2.   Leth A: Changes in plasma and extracellular fluid volumes in patients with essential hypertension during long-term treatment with hydrochlorothiazide. *Circulation* 1970;42:479-485.

3.   Unwin RJ, Ligueros M, Shakelton C, et al: Diuretics in the management of hypertension. In: Laragh JH, Brenner BM, eds. *Hypertension: Pathophysiology, Diagnosis, and Management*, 2nd ed. New York, Raven Press, 1995, pp 2785-2799.

4.   Siscovick DS, Raghunathan TE, Psaty BM, et al: Diuretic therapy for hypertension and the risk for primary cardiac arrest. *N Engl J Med* 1994;330:1852-1857.

5.   Hoes AW, Grobbee DE, Lufsen J, et al: Diuretics, β-blockers, and the risk for sudden cardiac death in hypertensive patients. *Ann Intern Med* 1995;123:481-487.

6.   Amery A, Berthoux P, Bulpitt C: Glucose intolerance during diuretic therapy. *Lancet* 1978;1:681-683.

7.   Weinberger MH: Antihypertensive therapy and lipids: evidence, mechanisms and implications. *Arch Intern Med* 1985;145:1102-1105.

8. Luft FC, Aronoff GR, Sloan RS, et al: Calcium channel blockade with nitrendipine. *Hypertension* 1985;7:438-442.

9. van Hamersvelt HW, Kloke HJ, de Jong DJ, et al: Oedema formation with the vasodilators nifedipine and diazoxide: direct local effect or sodium retention? *J Hypertens* 1996;14:1041-1046.

Chapter 7

Drug Therapy: Attacking Increased Resistance— Vasodilating Agents

Increased peripheral vascular resistance, primarily caused by vasoconstriction, is the hallmark of primary hypertension. Although this abnormality is not always the initial event in the pathogenesis of hypertension, vasoconstriction occurs as the blood pressure elevation becomes established. This may be the result of: (1) vascular 'remodeling' to resist the increased pressure with an alteration in the wall-to-lumen ratio; (2) increased vascular responsiveness to circulating or local vasopressor substances; or (3) the lack of vasodilatory substances such as kinins, vasodilator prostaglandins, or nitric oxide. Regardless of the mechanism, agents that induce vasorelaxation or vasodilation are effective in lowering blood pressure. With some of these agents, reflex physiologic responses, such as activation of the sympathetic nervous system by the baroreceptor mechanism or volume expansion from salt and water retention, may act to blunt their efficacy.

In general, the vasodilating drugs can be separated into two groups based on direct or indirect action on the vasculature through interference with one of the vasoconstrictor factors.

Direct-Acting Vasodilators

The prototype of this group of agents is sodium nitroprusside (Nipride). This very potent direct vasodilator requires intravenous administration and thus is reserved for the treatment of hypertensive urgencies and emergencies. It is administered by continuous intravenous drip while arterial pressure is constantly monitored so that the rate of administration can be titrated to the desired level of blood pressure reduction. Potent diuretics, which can be given intravenously if necessary, are typically required to combat the fluid retention that accompanies this agent. In addition, activation of the baroreceptor mechanism often requires administration of a β-blocker unless heart failure or other contraindications to the latter are present. Because it is a parenteral drug with the potential for thiocyanate toxicity, nitroprusside is used for short-term treatment. Simultaneous administration of an oral antihypertensive regimen is necessary after the patient's condition stabilizes so that the nitroprusside infusion can be discontinued. This is usually possible within 24 to 48 hours.

In the early 1950s, hydralazine (Apresoline®) became available for the treatment of hypertension. This agent acts to dilate precapillary arterioles and results in a marked decrease in peripheral vascular resistance. Hydralazine is relatively short-acting and generally must be taken 3 to 4 times daily to be effective in controlling blood pressure. Because of its rapid and short action, it typically stimulates the sympathetic nervous system via the baroreceptor mechanism, which results in a marked increase in pulse rate.[1] In patients with coronary artery disease, which is not uncommon in hypertensives, the combination of a rapid fall in blood pressure and a marked increase in heart rate can trigger myocardial ischemia and infarction. These effects can be blunted by administration of antisympathetic agents such as reserpine or, more recently, by β-adrenergic blocking drugs. Salt and water retention also occur with hydralazine, likely mediated by the marked stimulation of the renin-angiotensin-aldosterone system by this agent[1] so that potent diuretic agents are usually administered. This triple-therapy approach of reserpine, hydralazine, and a diuretic was popularized by the Veterans Administration Cooperative Study and even was produced as a single pill (Ser-Ap-Es®) by one pharmaceutical firm. The adverse effects associated with hydralazine, the need for multiple doses, and coadministration of diuretics and antisympathetic agents, coupled with the advent of equally effective newer drugs without these liabilities, has markedly reduced the use of hydralazine.

In the late 1970s, another direct-acting vasodilator, minoxidil (Loniten®), became available. This agent proved to be even more effective than hydralazine and was life-saving for many patients with severe refractory hypertension[2] before the availability of angiotensin-converting enzyme (ACE) inhibitors. Despite the potency of this agent, pseudotolerance caused by fluid retention and sympathetic activation limits its efficacy unless powerful doses of diuretics and β-blockers or antisympathetic drugs are also used. Minoxidil is also short-acting and requires multiple dosing for efficacy. With the advent of indirect-acting vasodilating agents, minoxidil has also been relegated to limited use. Characteristics and dosages of these agents are provided in Table 7-1.

Indirect-Acting Vasodilators

Peripheral α_1-Adrenergic Receptor Blockers

In the 1970s, prazosin (Minipress®) was introduced as the first of several agents (Table 7-1) to reduce blood pressure by blocking the actions of catecholamines on peripheral α_1-adrenergic receptors of vascular smooth muscle. Although this was an effective agent for the treatment of hypertension, the drug's use was diminished by its short duration of action, which required doses given 3 and 4 times a day, and by the pseudotolerance that occurred when the agent was given without a diuretic. A longer-acting agent, terazosin (Hytrin®), was more widely accepted, especially after some distinct advantages of the peripheral α_1-receptor blockers were recognized. These included a reduction in symptoms of benign prostatic hypertrophy, such as hesitancy and frequency of urination and nocturia, often experienced by older men with hypertension.[3] In addition, this class of drugs has been consistently shown to have beneficial effects on two major risk factors for cardiovascular disease often present with hypertension—insulin resistance-carbohydrate intolerance and dyslipidemia.[4,5] Alpha$_1$-blockers have also been shown to improve insulin sensitivity and carbohydrate tolerance in patients with diabetes and hypertension, and to lower triglycerides and total cholesterol while increasing high-density lipoproteins. The most recent drug of this group available for routine use is doxazosin (Cardura®), which has the longest duration of action in this class and is effective when given once a day. Doxazosin demonstrates all of the beneficial effects of the other agents of this group.[5]

Because the α_1-adrenergic receptors are involved in hemodynamic adjustments to changes in posture, administration of these agents can cause or exacerbate orthostatic hypotension in individuals predisposed to this problem. This is more common in the elderly and in those taking diuretic agents. Moreover, orthostatic hypotension is dose dependent, and is more likely to occur with the initial dose of α_1-blocker. For these reasons, it is recommended that treatment start with the lowest dose, that the initial dose be given at bedtime, and, if the patient is receiving a diuretic, that it be withdrawn for a day or two before beginning the α_1-blocker (if feasible). The drugs of this group may also cause drowsiness, but are generally well tolerated. At present, these agents receive greater attention because of their efficacy, safety, and beneficial effects on cardiovascular risk factors as well as on the symptoms of prostatism. Characteristics and dosages are shown in Table 7-1.

Table 7-1: Vasodilating Agents—Drugs, Duration, and Doses

Direct-Acting Vasodilators	Duration (h)
hydralazine (Apresoline®)	3-8
minoxidil (Loniten®)	12-18, 10-12

Indirect-Acting Vasodilators

α₁-adrenergic receptor blockers

doxazosin (Cardura®)	24
prazosin (Minipress®)	10
terazosin (Hytrin®)	24

Angiotensin-converting enzyme inhibitors

benazepril (Lotensin®)	24
captopril (Capoten®)	6, 8-12
enalapril (Vasotec®)	12-24
fosinopril (Monopril®)	24
lisinopril (Prinivil®, Zestril®)	24
moexipril (Univasc™)	24
perindopril (Aceon®)	24
quinapril (Accupril®)	12-24
ramipril (Altace®)	24
trandolapril (Mavik®)	24

Agents Interfering with the Renin-Angiotensin System

The introduction of ACE inhibitors ushered in a new era in antihypertensive therapy of drugs developed specifically for the effect on this important blood pressure-regulating system. These drugs were initially expected to have only a limited role for the treatment of most patients with hypertension. They were predicted to have the greatest use in conditions in which renin levels are usually elevated, such as malignant or accelerated forms of hypertension or in pa-

Doses (mg)	Frequency
25-100	t.i.d./q.i.d.
2.5-10	t.i.d./q.i.d.
1.0-16.0	q.d.
1.0-20.0	b.i.d./t.i.d.
1.0-10.0	q.d./b.i.d.
10-40	q.d.
12.5-200	t.i.d.
2.5-20	q.d./b.i.d.
10-40	q.d.
10-40	q.d.
7.5-30	q.d./b.i.d.
4-16	q.d./b.i.d.
20-80	q.d./b.i.d.
2.5-20	q.d.
1-8	q.d./b.i.d.

(continued on next page)

tients with renal vascular hypertension—situations that involve a minority of hypertensive patients. However, investigative studies demonstrated an impressive efficacy of ACE inhibitors across the entire spectrum of types of hypertension. Subsequent studies identified several possible mechanisms for blood pressure reduction with ACE inhibitors that did not involve the renin-angiotensin cascade, such as the bradykinin system and prostaglandins.[6]

Angiotensin-converting enzyme inhibitors also have several unique advantages over many other antihyperten-

Table 7-1: Vasodilating Agents—
Drugs, Duration, and Doses
(continued)

Indirect-acting vasodilators	Duration (h)
Angiotensin II receptor antagonists	
candesartan (Atacand®)	24
irbesartan (Avapro®)	24
losartan (Cozaar®)	24
telmisartan (Micardis®)	24
valsartan (Diovan®)	6-8, 24
Calcium channel entry blockers	
amlodipine (Norvasc®)	24-48
diltiazem (long-acting) (Cardizem® CD, Dilacor XR®, Tiazac™)	12-16
felodipine (Plendil® ER)	24
isradipine (DynaCirc®)	12
nicardipine (Cardene®)	3
nifedipine (long-acting) (Adalat® CC, Procardia XL®)	24
nisoldipine (Sular®)	24 (ER)
verapamil (long-acting) (Calan® SR, Covera® HS, Isoptin® SR, Verelan®)	14-18

sive agents. They improve insulin sensitivity and have no deleterious effects on lipids.[7] Moreover, when combined with diuretics, they demonstrate improved antihypertensive efficacy and either blunt or prevent many of the undesirable metabolic effects of diuretic therapy, such as hypokalemia, hyperglycemia, hyperlipidemia, and hyperuricemia.[8] Angiotensin-converting enzyme inhibitors have also demonstrated a protective effect in reducing the progression of diabetic renal disease.[9,10] This evidence is now sufficiently convincing to recommend the use of

Doses (mg)	Frequency
8-32	q.d.
75-300	q.d./b.i.d.
25-100	q.d./b.i.d.
40-160	q.d.
80-160	q.d.
2.5-10	q.d.
120-480	q.d.
2.5-10	q.d.
2.5-10	b.i.d.
60-120	t.i.d.
30-120	q.d.
10-40	q.d.
120-480	q.d.

ACE inhibitors for patients with diabetes, even in the face of normal blood pressure levels.[10] In addition, ACE inhibitors have been shown to reduce the progression of nondiabetic forms of renal disease. Important roles for ACE inhibitors have also been demonstrated in patients with congestive heart failure[11] and for the prevention of left ventricular enlargement and arrhythmias after myocardial infarction.[12] The major side effects of ACE inhibitors are a dry, nonproductive cough and skin rash. Rarely, angioedema is associated with this class of drugs, and is reported more often among African Americans than in other racial subgroups.

The major differences between the agents of this class are primarily in duration of action and frequency of administration, as indicated in Table 7-1. When ACE inhibitors are combined with other agents, such as diuretics or calcium channel entry blockers, the duration of antihypertensive action is often extended.

The renin-angiotensin system can also be blocked by the administration of an angiotensin II receptor blocker (ARB). ARBs have several advantages over ACE inhibitors. They have no apparent effect on bradykinin levels, which are typically increased by ACE inhibitors. It is thought that the bradykinin effect may account for some ACE inhibitor side effects, such as cough and angioedema, which are rare with ARBs. Drugs of the ARB class block activation of the AT_1 receptor responsible for vasoconstriction. They may also enhance vascular remodeling and thus prove to be beneficial in the treatment or prevention of some forms of cardiovascular disease. The prototype of this group of agents is represented by an analog of angiotensin II, saralasin (Sarenin), which requires intravenous administration, and thus has extremely limited use.[13] The first orally effective agent of this group, losartan (Cozaar®), is an antagonist of the AT_1 receptor thought to be responsible for the cardiovascular effects of angiotensin II.[14] This agent has no apparent effects on bradykinin, on other hormone receptors, or on ion channels. The typical dosage range is 25 to 100 mg taken once or twice daily. Although the experience with this agent is relatively recent, it appears to be well tolerated. Valsartan, irbesartan, candesartan, and telmisartan are the newest agents of this class to be marketed. The side effect profile observed in investigative studies suggests that symptoms such as skin rash, cough, respiratory infection, and sinusitis are less common with ARBs than with ACE inhibitors. The antihypertensive efficacy of this agent, like that of ACE inhibitors and other vasodilators, is enhanced when combined with small doses of diuretics. Several studies of ARBs are in progress to examine their usefulness in diabetic and other forms of renal disease, and in cardiovascular disorders, in addition to hypertension. Preliminary observations from these studies are most encouraging.

Calcium Channel Entry Blockers

Agents that induce vasodilation by preventing the entry of calcium into cells have been long favored both for the treatment of angina and for blood pressure reduction. These drugs appear to have the broadest efficacy of all of the antihypertensive agents, perhaps reflecting the importance of increased vascular resistance in the pathogenesis and maintenance of hypertension, independent of the initial abnormality. Increased intracellular calcium stores contribute to an enhanced response to vasoactive agents. Thus, reducing intracellular calcium by blocking entry via the slow calcium channel provides one approach to the treatment of hypertension that blunts the impact of vasoconstriction. As with the ACE inhibitors, this class of drugs has many representatives. However, they can be separated into three groups based on structure: the dihydropyridines (agents with generic names ending in —pine, such as amlodipine [Norvasc®], felodipine [Plendil® ER], and others listed in Table 7-1); the benzothiazepine or diltiazem group (Cardizem®, Dilacor XR®, Tiazac™); and the diphenylalkylamine-verapamil group (Calan® SR, Covera HS™, Isoptin®, and Verelan®). The characteristics and doses of these drugs are listed in Table 7-1. The major differences between the first three classes involve the relative affinities of their basic chemical structures for different vascular beds. For example, the dihydropyridines have the greatest affinity for the peripheral vasculature, and thus are the most potent antihypertensive and vasodilating agents. The diltiazem group has the greatest affinity for the coronary arteries, and are useful in angina in relatively low doses. Their antihypertensive effectiveness usually requires higher dosages, as shown in Table 7-1. Verapamil has the greatest effect on the cardiac conduction system and may cause bradycardia or delay atrioventricular (AV) conduction.

These classes of agents also differ in side effects. The dihydropyridines, because of their potency as peripheral vasodilators, are most likely to cause headache and flushing. This is particularly true of the short-acting agents that have a rapid and dramatic initial onset of action. In the past, immediate-release nifedipine was a favored drug for the treatment of urgent or emergent hypertension because it could rapidly lower elevated blood pressure.[15] However, this apparent virtue is now considered a liability with nifedipine because the blood pressure reduction is not only rapid and dramatic, but also uncontrolled and precipitous. This precipitous fall in pressure may have led to stroke and myocardial infarction in some patients treated with the short-acting, immediate-release preparations.[16] It also accounts for the marked activation of the sympathetic nervous system and the resultant tachycardia and increased myocardial oxygen demand that often occurs with the short-acting agents. In individuals with coronary artery disease, this could precipitate myocardial ischemia. Indeed, several recent reports implicated short-acting calcium channnel blockers of all three groups as associated with an increased risk of myocardial infarction.[17] Admittedly, these studies were retrospective and uncontrolled. Nonetheless, there is little, if any, justification for the use of the short-acting calcium channel entry blockers in view of both the adverse observations reported with them and the availability of other agents capable of lowering blood pressure in a slower or more controlled fashion without the adverse consequences. A long-term outcome study in older hypertensives (SYST-EUR) recently demonstrated a beneficial effect of the long-acting dihydropyridine calcium channel blocker nitrendipine (not available in the U.S.) in reducing cardiovascular events.[20] When completed, studies of treatment outcomes using the other longer-acting calcium channel blockers should provide information about the safety of these agents in broader groups of hypertensives using agents commonly prescribed in the United States.

The peripheral vasodilation of the calcium channel entry blockers, particularly the dihydropyridine group, also accounts for the reports of edema. This edema does not stem from excessive retention of salt and water, for these agents have an initial diuretic and natriuretic effect.[18] Rather, the edema results from intense capillary vasodilation, particularly of the precapillary vessels. This increases capillary pressure; fluid escapes from the vasculature, and it settles in the most dependent tissues.[19] This edema is managed with occasional elevation of the legs, with the use of elasticized stockings, or, in severe cases, with the addition of a small dose of an ACE inhibitor that dilates the postcapillary arteriole and reduces capillary pressure. Diuretics are generally *not* required to treat the edema associated with calcium channel entry blocker therapy.

Diltiazem is associated with edema, but it occurs much less often than with the dihydropyridine agents. However, diltiazem can cause headache, nasal stuffiness, skin rash, cough, and constipation. Constipation is most often reported with verapamil in its various forms. Verapamil can also cause bradycardia and heart block, and should be given cautiously in patients treated with digitalis preparations.

It is important to recognize the unique 'packaging' of some of the calcium channel entry blockers. For example, while felodipine (Plendil® ER) is an extended-release tablet, Dilacor XR® is an extended-release capsule that contains various numbers (2, 3, or 4) of 60-mg extended-release diltiazem. Verelan® contains sustained-release pellets of verapamil in a gelatin capsule. Procardia XL® is a minipump consisting of an insoluble, nondegradable cover with a laser-drilled aperture capable of absorbing water from the gastrointestinal tract, which then expands the filler layer of the tablet and diffuses the immediate-release nifedipine out of the tablet as it transits the gastrointestinal tract. Thus, the tablet can be recovered, apparently intact, from the stool, but the nifedipine has been dissipated. For these reasons, patients should be instructed about the unusual nature of the products and told not to attempt to cut them. Another recent innovation in the delivery of calcium channel entry blockers is the formulation of verapamil in a variation of the minipump described above and known as Covera HS™. In this form, verapamil is in the active layer of the push-pull mechanism, but the outer nondegradable layer is covered with a time-release coating that requires 5 to 6 hours for dissolution. The preparation is taken at bedtime so that the active verapamil begins to enter the system about 1 to 2 hours before the patient awakens, thus providing protection against the cardiovascular surges of the early morning hours, when cardiovascular events such as angina, myocardial infarction, and sudden death are increased.

References

1.   Lees KR, Reid JL: The pharmacology of antihypertensive drugs and drug-drug interactions. In: Laragh JH, Brenner BM, eds. *Hypertension: Pathophysiology, Diagnosis, and Management*, 2nd ed. New York, Raven Press, 1995, pp 2985-2995.

2.   Pettinger WA: Minoxidil and the treatment of severe hypertension. *N Engl J Med* 1980;303:922-926.

3.   Hedlund H, Andersson KE, Ek AK: Effects of prazosin in patients with benign prostatic obstruction. *J Urol* 1983;130:275-278.

4.   Weinberger MH: Antihypertensive therapy and lipids: evidence, mechanisms and implications. *Arch Intern Med* 1985;145: 1102-1105.

5.   Dominguez LJ, Weinberger MH, Cefalu WT, et al: Doxazosin improves insulin sensitivity and lowers blood pressure in type II diabetic hypertensives with no changes in tyrosine kinase activity or insulin binding. *Am J Hypertens* 1995;8:528-532.

6.   Waeber B, Nussberger J, Brunner HR: Angiotensin-converting enzyme inhibitors in hypertension. In: Laragh JH, Brenner

BM, eds. *Hypertension: Pathophysiology, Diagnosis, and Management,* 2nd ed. New York, Raven Press, 1995, pp 2861-2875.

7.   Pollare T, Lithell H, Berne C: A comparison of the effects of hydrochlorothiazide and captopril on glucose and lipid metabolism. *N Engl J Med* 1989;321:868-873.

8.   Weinberger MH: Influence of an angiotensin-converting enzyme inhibitor on diuretic-induced metabolic effects in hypertension. *Hypertension* 1983;5:132-138.

9.   Lewis EJ, Hunsicker LG, Pain RP, et al: The effect of angiotensin-converting enzyme inhibition on diabetic nephropathy. *N Engl J Med* 1993;329:1456-1462.

10.   Ravid M, Savin H, Jutrin I, et al: Long-term stabilizing effect of angiotensin-converting enzyme inhibition on plasma creatinine and on proteinuria in normotensive type II diabetic patients. *Ann Intern Med* 1993;118:577-581.

11.   Deedwania PC: Angiotensin-converting enzyme inhibitors in congestive heart failure. *Arch Intern Med* 1990;150:1798-1805.

12.   Gavras H, Gavras I: Cardioprotective potential of angiotensin converting enzyme inhibitors. *Hypertension* 1991;9:385-392.

13.   Pals DT, Denning GS Jr, Keenen RE: Historical development of saralasin. *Kidney Int* 1979;59:S7-S10.

14.   Timmermans PBMWM, Carini DJ, Chiu AT, et al: The discovery of a new class of highly specific nonpeptide angiotensin II receptor antagonists. *Am J Hypertens* 1991;4:275S-281S.

15.   Kiowski W, Bertel O, Erne P, et al: Haemodynamic and reflex mechanism of acute and chronic antihypertensive therapy with the calcium channel blocker nifedipine. *Hypertension* 1983; 5:170-174.

16.   Furberg CD, Psaty BM, Meyer JV: Nifedipine: dose-related increase in mortality in patients with coronary heart disease. *Circulation* 1995;92:1326-1331.

17.   Psaty BM, Heckert SR, Koepsell TD, et al: The risk of myocardial infarction associated with antihypertensive drug therapies *JAMA* 1995;274:620-625.

18.   Luft FC, Aronoff Gr, Sloan RS, et al: Calcium channel blockade with nitrendipine. *Hypertension* 1985;7:438-442.

19. van Hamersvelt HW, Kloke HJ, de Jong DJ, et al: Oedema formation with the vasodilators nifedipine and diazoxide: direct local effect or sodium retention? *J Hypertens* 1996;14:1041-1046

20. Staessen JA, Fagard R, Thijs L, et al, for the Systolic Hypertension-Europe (SYST-EUR) Trial Investigators: Morbidity and mortality in the placebo-controlled European Trial on Isolated Systolic Hypertension in the Elderly. *Lancet* 1997;360:757-764.

Chapter 8

Drug Therapy: Antisympathetic Agents

The sympathetic nervous system has long been recognized as a modulator of blood pressure. Evidence suggests that the etiology of blood pressure elevation in some individuals is related to enhanced sympathetic nervous system activity or to vascular response. Physical clues to enhanced sympathetic activity include a hyperdynamic chest wall or resting tachycardia. Thus, it is not surprising that drugs that attack the sympathetic nervous system would be useful in the treatment of hypertension. In the era before such agents were available, lumbar sympathectomy was transiently effective in reducing markedly elevated blood pressure. This was followed by the use of ganglionic blocking agents such as hexamethonium, or agents capable of diminishing the peripheral vascular effects of sympathetic discharge, such as the Veratrum alkaloids. Because of the severity and frequency of their side effects, these agents were soon abandoned in favor of newer drugs that had equivalent or improved efficacy and were better tolerated. This chapter reviews these agents based on their sites of action (Table 8-1).

Central α_2-Agonists

Stimulation of central α_2-adrenergic sites causes a decrease in central sympathetic outflow, thereby reducing peripheral sympathetic tone. One of the early agents available

Table 8-1: Antisympathetic Agents: Drugs and Dosages

	Doses (mg/d)	Frequency
central α_2-agonists		
α-methyldopa (Aldomet®)	250-2000	t.i.d./q.i.d.
clonidine (Catapres®)	0.2-2.0	b.i.d.
clonidine patch (TTS®)	0.1-0.3	weekly
guanabenz (Wytensin®)	4-32	b.i.d.
guanfacine (Tenex®)	1-4	q.d.
peripheral antagonists		
reserpine	0.1-0.25	q.d.
α- and ß-adrenergic receptor blockers		
carvedilol (Coreg®)	3.125-25	b.i.d.
labetalol (Trandate®, Normodyne®)	200-1200	b.i.d.
ß-adrenergic receptor blockers		
cardioselective (β_1) blockers (dose dependent)		
*acetbutolol (Sectral®)	400-1200	q.d./b.i.d.
atenolol (Tenormin®)	25-200	q.d./b.i.d.
betaxolol (Kerlone®)	10-40	q.d.
bisoprolol (Zebeta®)	5-20	q.d.
metoprolol (Lopressor®)	100-450	b.i.d.
metoprolol XL (Toprol XL®)	50-200	q.d.

*Indicates β-blockers with intrinsic sympathomimetic activity (ISA).

(continued on next page)

for the treatment of hypertension, α-methyldopa (Aldomet®), appears to act in this fashion as well as serving as a false neurotransmitter at the peripheral sympathetic synapses. The major limitations of this agent have been the frequency of administration required for smooth blood

Table 8-1: Antisympathetic Agents: Drugs and Dosages *(continued)*

	Doses (mg/d)	Frequency
nonselective (β_1,β_2) blockers		
*carteolol (Cartrol®)	2.5-10	q.d.
nadolol (Corgard)	40-160	q.d.
penbutolol (Levatol®)	10-40	q.d./b.i.d.
*pindolol (Visken®)	5-60	b.i.d./t.i.d.
propranolol (Inderal®)	40-480	t.i.d./q.i.d.
propranolol (Inderal® LA)	60-640	q.d.
timolol (Blocadren®)	20-120	b.i.d./t.i.d.
ganglionic blockers		
guanadrel (Hylorel®)	10-75	b.i.d.
guanethidine (Ismelin®)	10-100	q.d.

*Indicates β-blockers with intrinsic sympathomimetic activity (ISA).

pressure control and the side effects associated with its use. Lethargy and sexual dysfunction, reflecting the central action, are common. Orthostatic hypotension, hemolytic anemia, and hepatitis occur less often.

A group of newer drugs with a similar central mechanism of action includes clonidine (Catapres®, in both oral and transdermal forms), guanabenz (Wytensin®), and guanfacine (Tenex®). All of these agents share similar side effects of lethargy and nasal congestion. Because clonidine and guanabenz require twice-daily dosing, the second dose should be taken near bedtime. In addition, if the total dose is above the starting level, a larger dose can be given at bedtime than in the morning to minimize the central side effects while maintaining antihypertensive efficacy. Abrupt withdrawal or discontinuation of these agents has occasionally been associated with rebound hypertension. This can be avoided by gradual withdrawal or by tapering the dose. It occurs more commonly with higher doses of the drugs (ie, >0.6 mg/d).

The transdermal form of clonidine is a unique antihypertensive drug administration system. The entry of drug from the patch is slow, as is its onset and offset of action. It takes at least one day to reach steady-state levels. This formulation is particularly useful for patients who are unable to take oral medication and for antihypertensive coverage during the perioperative period. In the latter, it is important to bear in mind that the patch must be applied 24 to 48 hours *before* surgery to obtain optimal efficacy.

Peripheral Antiadrenergic Agents

The sympathetic nervous system is more commonly attacked at the peripheral level. The peripheral α_1-adrenergic receptor blockers, which indirectly lower blood pressure by reducing catecholamine-induced vasoconstriction, are reviewed in Chapter 7. Reserpine, a derivative of the Veratrum alkaloids, acts to lower blood pressure by inhibiting peripheral sympathetic tone. This agent is not often used today because it can result in lethargy, depression, sexual dysfunction, nasal stuffiness, and gastric ulceration.

Combined Alpha-Adrenergic and Beta-Adrenergic Receptor Blockade

Labetalol (Normodyne®, Trandate®) is a combined peripheral α-adrenergic and β-adrenergic receptor blocker. As with the peripheral α-receptor blockers, orthostatic hypotension may occur with labetalol. Dizziness, fatigue, gastrointestinal symptoms, nasal stuffiness, and sexual dysfunction are more common side effects with this agent. Because of the likelihood of side effects, this agent is usually reserved for second- or third-step therapy for most patients with hypertension, rather than as the initial treatment. Carvedilol (Coreg®) has been approved by the Food and Drug Administration (FDA) for the treatment of hypertension and congestive heart failure.

Peripheral Beta-Adrenergic Receptor Blockers

The peripheral β-adrenergic receptor blocking agents have been enthusiastically used for more than 20 years. A large number of these agents are available throughout the world. The drugs listed in Table 8-1 represent those approved for treatment of hypertension in the United States, and are separated on the basis of cardioselectivity and intrinsic sympathomimetic activity (ISA). Cardioselectivity refers to the preferential effect of a β-blocker to occupy the β_1-receptor, governing adrenergic effects to stimulate the heart, rather than the β_2-receptor, which has a greater effect on dilatation of smooth muscle of the bronchus and peripheral vasculature. It is important to realize that cardioselectivity is a *relative* rather than an absolute phenomenon, and that it is dose dependent. Thus, the peripheral vasoconstriction, decreased blood flow, and bronchospasm that characterize nonselective β-blockers may also occur with the cardioselective agents when they are used in sufficiently high doses to block the β_2-receptor.[1] Unfortunately, one of the distinct advantages of β-blockers—their cardioprotective effect in the primary or secondary prevention of myocardial infarction—requires the use of high enough doses to make the advantage of cardioselectivity negligible. In the lower range of antihypertensive doses, however, fewer side effects attributable to β_2-blockade occur with the cardioselective drugs.

Beta-adrenergic blocking agents lower blood pressure primarily by their effects on the β_1-receptor to decrease cardiac output by reducing both heart rate and contractility.[1] A good index of the efficacy of a given dose of β-blocker is the reduction in heart rate. This can also be a useful clue regarding patient compliance or evidence of difficulty with absorption or metabolism of the drug. Unfortunately, the decrease in heart rate, cardiac output, and blood pressure also contribute to the lassitude that patients often experience. Recent observations indicate that β-blockers may be beneficial in some patients with congestive heart failure. In addition, the combined α_1 and β-blocker carvedilol (Coreg®) has been found to be effective in congestive heart failure.

Beta-blockers are useful in the treatment of angina pectoris because the reduction in heart rate, contractility, and blood pressure results in reduced myocardial oxygen demand. They should be used with caution in insulin-requiring diabetics because they mask the symptoms of hypoglycemia that are catecholamine dependent.

Beta-blockers have a variety of metabolic effects that may be a disadvantage in many patients with hypertension. These agents worsen insulin sensitivity and thus can precipitate or worsen carbohydrate intolerance and diabetes.[2] They also have a consistent adverse impact on the lipid profile by increasing triglycerides and total cholesterol and lowering high-density lipoprotein (HDL).[3] Although small, these lipid changes persist for the duration of treatment, rather than being transient. This finding is based on improvement in the lipid profile after cessation of the β-blocker. This is not surprising because α-adrenergic receptor blockers have exactly the opposite effect (see Chapter 7), and because catecholamines are known to be involved in lipoprotein synthesis and/or metabolism. These metabolic effects of β-blockers are not seen with the combined α-β blocker labetalol, or with the β-blockers possessing ISA.[3]

The ISA agents, indicated by asterisks in Table 8-1, act as partial agonists of the β-receptor and, thus, insulin resistance and dyslipidemia are uncommon. However, these agents have not been shown to have cardioprotective effects, which have been observed with the β-blockers lacking ISA.

Ganglionic Blocking Drugs

The ganglionic blocking agents (Table 8-1) lower blood pressure by inhibiting norepinephrine release from nerve endings during sympathetic stimulation, and by depleting neuronal stores of norepinephrine. These drugs typically are associated with orthostatic hypotension, increased heart rate, fluid retention, diarrhea, and retrograde ejaculation or impotence in men. They should not be used in patients receiving monoamine oxidase (MAO) inhibitors. The use of sympathomimetic agents, such as those found in over-the-counter cold remedies, decongestants, and diet suppressants, by patients concurrently taking ganglionic blockers can cause precipitous increases in blood pressure. Physicians may not be aware of the common use (and abuse) of over-the-counter or sympathomimetic agents by patients. This, coupled with the side effects of the ganglionic blockers, have generally reserved them for use in refractory patients as third- or fourth-level therapy.

References

1. Prichard BN, Cruikshank JM: Beta blockade in hypertension: past present and future. In: Laragh JH, Brenner BM, eds. *Hypertension: Pathophysiology, Diagnosis, and Management*, 2nd ed. New York, Raven Press, 1995, pp 2827-2859.

2. Joint National Committee on Prevention, Detection, Evaluation and Treatment of High Blood Pressure (JNC V). *Arch Intern Med* 1997;157:2413-2446.

3. Weinberger MH: Antihypertensive therapy and lipids: evidence, mechanisms and implications. *Arch Intern Med* 1985;145: 1102-1105.

Chapter 9

Hypertension Associated With Other Disorders and Cardiovascular Disease Risk Factors

Most patients with hypertension have other medical problems or risk factors that may interact with blood pressure or may influence the choice of antihypertensive therapy. Elevated blood pressure is often associated with insulin resistance, carbohydrate sensitivity, frank diabetes mellitus, or dyslipidemia.[1,2] The manifestations may include elevated triglycerides, elevated total cholesterol, or reduced high-density lipoprotein (HDL). The constellation of obesity, dyslipidemia, carbohydrate intolerance, and hypertension is sometimes designated as *Syndrome X* or the *metabolic syndrome*.[3] It is not the only metabolic abnormality found in patients with hypertension, however. Some patients may have hyperuricemia, which is also associated with an increased risk of coronary artery disease. Renal disease is also common. It is often difficult to discern whether the renal disease precedes the blood pressure elevation or results from long-standing, inadequately treated hypertension.

Echocardiographic studies have indicated that a substantial number of patients with hypertension have evidence of left ventricular hypertrophy (LVH).[4] Because this finding is based on the more sensitive echocardiogram, it has heightened concern about LVH as a risk factor for cardiovascular disease, which is less likely to be identified by electrocardiogram or chest x-ray. Many patients with hypertension also have coronary artery disease, demonstrated by a history of myocardial infarction or angina. Congestive heart failure and arrhythmias may occur more often in hypertensives than in the normotensive population. Stroke, transient ischemic attacks (TIAs), and peripheral vascular disease are also common, as are pulmonary problems, which range from asthmatic bronchitis to obstructive airway disease and emphysema. Because the prevalence of hypertension increases with age, the disorders of older patients, such as arthritis, depression, prostatic enlargement, and sexual dysfunction, often occur with elevated blood pressure. This chapter addresses the considerations posed when these problems are seen in a patient with hypertension.

Metabolic Abnormalities

Frank diabetes mellitus, typically the noninsulin-dependent, maturity-onset form, is often found in the hypertensive population. Studies have recently provided evidence of a more subtle abnormality of carbohydrate metabolism in many patients with hypertension.[1,5] Insulin resistance has been shown to occur in hypertensive patients who demonstrate no evidence of diabetes.[5] Although this finding is more common in obese patients with hypertension, it has also been found in hypertensives of lean body mass. The mechanism for this abnormality is under investigation, but preliminary evidence suggests that the impairment of tissue response to insulin (insulin resistance) may partially result from the hemodynamic consequences of hypertension.[6] Vasoconstriction of the muscle bed can reduce the effectiveness of insulin by a mass action effect. In addition, evidence indicates that this may be related to deficient production of nitric oxide, a potent vasodilator.[6]

For patients who are obese, weight loss and exercise often lead to improvement of insulin resistance.[7] In the evaluation of a hypertensive patient, measurement of blood glucose is a requisite and, in those individuals with elevated fasting values, additional studies are recommended, such as plasma insulin-to-glucose ratios, 2-hour postglucose blood sugar, or glucose tolerance tests. In addition to baseline observations, follow-up studies after initiation of antihypertensive therapy may also be appropriate because many of these agents may influence the action of insulin.

Some antihypertensive agents, such as β-adrenergic blockers and diuretics, can worsen insulin sensitivity and should be used cautiously, if at all, in hypertensive patients with abnormalities of carbohydrate metabolism.[8] In addition, β-blockers are relatively contraindicated in insulin-requiring diabetics because of the potential to mask or prevent recognition of the symptoms of hypoglycemia. In contrast to these antihypertensive agents that worsen insulin sensitivity, several can enhance the effectiveness of insulin and are preferred in patients with carbohydrate intolerance. The peripheral α_1-receptor antagonists, prazosin (Minipress®), terazosin (Hytrin®), and doxazosin (Cardura®), have been shown to improve insulin sensitivity, as have the angiotensin-converting enzyme (ACE) inhibitors.[8,9] Although evidence is not yet available on the effect of angiotensin II receptor blockers (ARBs) on insulin sensitivity, studies should soon provide this information. The other antihypertensive drugs either have not been carefully evaluated for their effects on insulin action, or are essentially neutral in this regard.

Dyslipidemia is another common metabolic abnormality in patients with hypertension.[2] Recent observations indicate that this is a major risk factor for cardiovascular disease; that the concurrence of both dyslipidemia and hypertension have a combined impact on this risk; and that even small changes in lipids can have a dramatic effect on these events. Dyslipidemia may present as an elevation of total cholesterol or triglycerides (also shown to be a risk factor for vascular disease), or with reduced levels of HDL. Measurement of these lipid components then permits calculation of the atherogenic low-density lipoprotein (LDL) fraction, which can also be measured directly. Thus, baseline measurement of the entire lipid profile is an important part of the evaluation of hypertension and should be repeated annually, which is particularly true in view of the effects of several antihypertensive drugs on lipid and lipoprotein fractions.[10]

Not all of the LDL particles are equally atherogenic. The small, dense LDL appears to be the main factor, but practical clinical measurement of this component is not yet possible. Some investigators recommend using the total cholesterol-to-HDL ratio, because it is a more useful way to assess atherogenic risk than any of the individual lipid measurements. When this ratio is less than 3.0, the cardio-vascular risk is considered low, unless the HDL value is abnormal. A ratio above 5.0 indicates the need for aggressive intervention. In the intermediate range, decisions about treatment depend on assessment of other risk factors and on family history. Lipoprotein(a) has been identified as a marker of atherogenic risk but is not routinely measured, nor are any interventions now available to alter its level. Future studies may provide more information on this major component of vascular disease.

Doses of diuretics that are effective in lowering blood pressure when used as monotherapy also raise total cholesterol and triglycerides.[10] This is true for all diuretic agents, including indapamide (Lozol®), furosemide (Lasix®), torsemide (Demadex®), and others when used at full anti-hypertensive doses. Moreover, these lipid effects do not dissipate with time, but are found to decrease when the agents are withdrawn. Beta-adrenergic blocking drugs, including both β_1 (cardioselective) and $\beta_1\beta_2$ (nonselective) agents, increase triglycerides and reduce HDL.[10]

In contrast to the adverse effects of diuretics and β-blockers on lipids, the peripheral α_1-blockers have demonstrated a beneficial effect by reducing triglycerides and total cholesterol and by raising HDL.[10] These opposing effects of α-adrenergic and β-adrenergic blocking drugs on the lipid profile are consistent with the known role for catecholamines in lipid synthesis and metabolism. Data indicate that other antihypertensive agents have a neutral effect on lipids or have not been adequately evaluated.

Hyperuricemia is another metabolic abnormality occasionally observed in patients with hypertension. In recent epidemiologic surveys, hyperuricemia has been associated with cardiovascular disease, particularly myocardial infarction. No mechanisms have been elucidated to explain the connection between uric acid and vascular disease, nor is it known whether intervention alters this relationship. Nonetheless, awareness of this finding and assessment of uric acid levels are appropriate during the evaluation of a hypertensive patient. Because diuretics can significantly increase uric acid levels and provoke acute attacks of gout, they should be used with caution, if at all, in patients with hyperuricemia or a history of gout. Most other antihypertensive agents have no apparent effect on uric acid, with two exceptions. First, the angiotensin-converting enzyme (ACE) inhibitors are known to reduce uric acid levels in hyperuricemic patients,[11] which appears to be related to the effects of angiotensin II on tubular reabsorption or secretion of urate. The second exception is the ARBs, which also demonstrate this effect.[12] These agents may be preferred in patients with known hyperuricemia or gout. Finally, the combination of an ACE inhibitor with a diuretic has been shown to blunt or prevent the adverse diuretic effects on potassium loss, hypercholesterolemia, hyperglycemia, and hyperuricemia. This combination may be the therapeutic choice for diuretic treatment in a hypertensive patient with one or more of these risk factors.

Renal Disease

As previously mentioned, when renal impairment is detected in patients with hypertension, it is not usually clear whether the renal disease precedes the development of hypertension, or if it results from inadequately treated blood pressure elevation. The patient's history may occasionally provide a clue, but specific tests are usually required to rule out renal vascular disease or other renal causes of hypertension. If no remediable etiology can be identified, then attention should be directed to the treatment of hypertension, with special consideration for the preservation of renal function. Several therapeutic approaches may be effective because the blood pressure elevation associated with renal disease may result from a reduced capacity to excrete salt and water (volume expansion and salt sensitivity), from increased production of vasoconstrictor factors such as renin, or, most often, from a combination of these factors. Although diuretic treatment is important, it must be recalled that the response to the proximal-tubule thiazide agents is diminished in the face of renal impairment (serum creatinine ≥1.8 mg/dL). Thus, loop diuretics are often required. Excessive volume depletion, however, further decreases renal function and, therefore, monitoring renal function and blood pressure response is important to determine the optimal dosage and frequency of these medications. Vasodilators can also optimize renal blood flow and lower blood pressure by attacking the vasoconstrictor component. Angiotensin-converting enzyme inhibitors (and ARBs) appear to be ideal choices in this regard. When hypertension and renal impairment result from collagen vascular disease, such as systemic lupus erythematosus, scleroderma, and periarteritis nodosa, increased renin production generally occurs. In these settings, ACE inhibitors have been very effective both in lowering the blood pressure and in improving renal function. However, as noted in the review of renal vascular hypertension (see Chapter 4), deterioration of renal function may occur with these agents when the drive for glomerular filtration is primarily maintained by intrarenal angiotensin II-induced efferent arteriolar constriction. Thus, careful follow-up of renal function is required when these agents are used in patients with known renal impairment.

Proteinuria is often found in association with hypertension when renal involvement is present, and has been associated with an increased risk of cardiovascular disease.[13] Researchers have suggested that some calcium channel entry blockers may increase the magnitude of proteinuria, which requires careful follow-up.[14]

Cardiac and Peripheral Vascular Disorders

Cardiac problems such as LVH are common in patients with hypertension.[4] This is a major risk factor for myocardial infarction, presumably by adversely affecting the supply-demand relationship between coronary blood flow and myocardial oxygen requirements. Coronary reserve is diminished in the presence of LVH, which predisposes patients to arrhythmias, particularly in the presence of hypokalemia, and is a major risk factor for congestive heart failure. For all of these reasons, prevention or reduction of LVH is desirable. Regression of the thickened ventricle usually occurs with blood pressure reduction, and limited evidence suggests that this may reduce the adverse effects associated with LVH. It is clear that not all antihypertensive agents have equal effects in inducing regression of LVH, although blood pressure reduction is generally helpful.[15] The known influences of various antihypertensives on the development of ventricular hypertrophy may provide clues to their possible differential effects. Catecholamines (acting via adrenergic receptors) and angiotensin II are significantly involved. Thus, it is not surprising that agents interfering with these factors have been consistently shown to induce regression of LVH, including ACE inhibitors (and presumably ARBs, for which evidence is currently experimental), peripheral α_1-receptor blockers, β-blockers *without* ISA, calcium channel entry blockers, and diuretics.[15] Drugs capable of markedly stimulating the renin-angiotensin and catecholamine systems, such as hydralazine and minoxidil, are not consistently associated with regression of LVH. Centrally acting α-agonists have not been carefully studied for their effects on hypertrophy.

Another manifestation of heart disease in patients with hypertension is angina pectoris. This results from an aberration in the relationship between myocardial oxygen requirements and supply (coronary perfusion). Agents that increase coronary blood flow or reduce oxygen demand should have a beneficial effect on angina. Beta-blocking drugs without ISA decrease myocardial oxygen demand by reducing heart rate, contractility, and blood pressure, as do the calcium channel entry blockers that lower heart rate, such as diltiazem (Cardizem®, Dilacor XR®, Tiazac™) and verapamil (Calan® SR, Covera™, Isoptin®, Verelan®). In addition, all of the long-acting calcium channel blockers, including the dihydropyridines and the two groups listed above, increase coronary blood flow. However, short-acting calcium channel blockers that stimulate sympathetic nervous system activity by a reflex mechanism, and thus increase heart rate and myocardial contractility, may actually have an adverse effect on myocardial oxygen demand and perfusion.[16] Similarly, direct-acting vasodilators such as hydralazine and minoxidil have been associated with worsening of angina and provocation of acute myocardial infarction by markedly stimulating catecholamines, and thus heart rate.

Hypertension and LVH are major risk factors for the development of congestive heart failure. As the myocardium fails, blood pressure often falls; the systemic response to a decrease in cardiac output then activates the pressor systems in an attempt to improve blood flow. Thus, increased levels of renin, angiotensin II, and catecholamines are typical in heart failure.[17] This reduces tissue perfusion and further increases the myocardial load to induce a vicious circle. Diuretic administration is useful to attempt to decrease fluid retention, but this beneficial effect is often blunted by the increase in renin and catecholamines induced by volume depletion. In recent years, the beneficial effects of vasodilator therapy in congestive heart failure have been demonstrated, and ACE inhibitors have been the most effective of these agents, not only in providing symptomatic improvement, but also in extending life span.[18] It is likely that the angiotensin II receptor antagonists will also have this beneficial effect on congestive heart failure. Evidence also suggests that ACE inhibitors can reduce the risk of sudden death during or after acute myocardial infarction, and that their administration reduces the likelihood of ventricular enlargement, subsequent congestive heart failure, and reinfarction.[19]

Cardiac arrhythmias also occur frequently in patients with hypertension, and can range in effect from innocuous to life-threatening. There may be different mechanisms involved in the arrhythmogenesis in hypertension. The role of LVH has already been mentioned, and myocardial ischemia, catecholamine stimulation, and electrolyte abnormalities may also be involved. Several recent reports indicate that hypertensive patients who receive diuretics without potassium supplementation or potassium-sparing agents, and those who take β-adrenergic blocking drugs, are at increased risk of sudden death.[20,21] It is not yet clearly established that specific treatments for hypertension are capable of reducing arrhythmias and sudden death, but some general observations may provide an intuitive basis for approaching this issue. For example, avoiding potassium and magnesium depletion is obvious. Therapeutic approaches designed to reduce LVH would also be appropriate, as would minimizing or blocking the effects of the increase in catecholamines and angiotensin II. Finally, reducing myocardial oxygen demand may also be beneficial, although the epidemiologic association of sudden death with β-blocker therapy is confusing on this issue.

Patients with cerebral vascular disease should avoid dehydration and marked hypotension, particularly with postural change. Unless otherwise contraindicated, most patients with hypertension should also receive small doses

(81 mg/d) of aspirin to reduce the likelihood of thrombosis. Smooth and adequate blood pressure control is another important factor in preventing recurrence of cerebral vascular disease. The symptoms of peripheral vascular disease can be made worse by an increase in blood viscosity (often associated with diuretic therapy) and by the use of β-blocking agents, particularly of the nonselective group. Calcium channel entry blockers, other vasodilators, and agents such as pentoxifylline (Trental®) may relieve symptoms of peripheral vascular disease.

Pulmonary Disease, Arthritis, Prostatism, Sexual Function, and Depression

A history of bronchial asthma, evidence of obstructive lung disease, or emphysema may influence therapeutic choices for hypertension. In general, β-adrenergic blocking drugs should be avoided in such patients if possible, because of the tendency of these agents to precipitate bronchospasm by blocking the β_2-receptor of bronchial smooth muscle.[22] The use of cardioselective (β_1) blockers can be attempted in some cases but, as mentioned in Chapter 8, the selectivity of these agents for the different β-receptors is dose dependent, and is often lost at the doses necessary for blood pressure control. Another class of drugs that may not be ideal in patients with pulmonary disease is the ACE inhibitor group. Although these agents do not induce bronchial spasm, they often cause a persistent, dry cough that may exacerbate impaired pulmonary function, and may be related to the action of this class of drugs to alter the degradation of bradykinin. Because kinins mediate the response to inflammatory stimuli, this is a feasible explanation. If true, one would predict that drugs interfering with the renin-angiotensin system by a mechanism other than ACE inhibition might not have such effects. This appears to be the case with the angiotensin II receptor antagonists, which provide antihypertensive efficacy comparable with that of ACE inhibitors without the common side effect of cough.

Because most patients with hypertension are among the older population in whom arthritis is common, treatment of this disorder must also be considered carefully. Nonsteroidal anti-inflammatory drugs (NSAIDs) are known to promote salt and water retention by the kidneys because of their effects on renal tubular function. In addition, they can worsen renal function. Because both of these factors may be concerns for hypertensive patients, NSAIDs should be used cautiously and only when other analgesic approaches to arthritis, such as aspirin and acetaminophen are ineffective. The NSAIDs also prevent or blunt the effectiveness of many antihypertensive agents, including diuretics, β-blockers, and ACE inhibitors.[23] Because of their fluid-retaining and potassium-losing characteristics, corticosteroids should be used cautiously in patients with hypertension. When the use of corticosteroids becomes necessary, renal function, electrolytes, and blood pressure must be monitored carefully. If blood pressure becomes elevated during corticosteroid treatment, diuretic therapy should be considered with careful attention to potassium levels.

Benign prostatic hyperplasia (BPH) is also common among hypertensive men. Symptoms of urinary hesitancy, frequency, dysuria, and nocturia can often be improved by administration of peripheral α_1-receptor blockers such as prazosin (Minipress®), terazosin (Hytrin®), and doxazosin (Cardura®). It is not clear whether there is an additive effect on urinary symptoms when α_1-receptor blockers are combined with 5α-reductase inhibitors such as finasteride (Proscar®) for BPH.

Impairment of sexual function is common in men with hypertension. Moreover, the problem is often compounded by drugs used for blood pressure reduction. Atherosclerosis, common in hypertensive men, reduces perfusion, as can the reduction of blood pressure itself. Both diuretics and drugs that interfere with sympathetic nervous system function have classically been associated with worsening of sexual function in men. In relative terms, the antihypertensive agents reported least likely to cause or worsen sexual function have been the peripheral α_1-receptor blockers, the ACE inhibitors, and the calcium channel entry blockers. There is inadequate experience with the ARBs to comment on their effect on sexual function.

Some pharmacologic approaches are occasionally helpful in sexual dysfunction. Papaverine (Pavabid®) 150 to 300 mg b.i.d., or yohimbine (Yocon®) 5.4 mg t.i.d., or sildenafil (Viagra®) 25 to 100 mg/d may improve sexual function for some men. Alprostadil (Caverject®) is available for direct injection into the corpus cavernosum or by instillation *per urethra*. If primary testicular failure is present, as evidenced by suppressed plasma testosterone levels, administration of testosterone replacement in oral or parenteral forms may be helpful. When these efforts fail, consultation with a urologist who has special expertise in sexual function is usually indicated.

Very little is known about the effects of various forms of antihypertensive therapy on sexual function in women. Such information has been hampered by the difficulty in developing objective parameters for assessing this problem in women and by the difficulty in validating questionnaires used for this purpose.

Depression also occurs more often in the older population. In addition, the central nervous system actions of many antihypertensive agents could affect this problem. Reserpine has long been associated with depression, as has α-methyldopa (Aldomet®), which has a similar mechanism of action. Curiously, the centrally acting α_2-agonists have not been implicated in depression as frequently as reserpine and α-methyldopa. Beta-blockers have also been associated with depression. It has been suggested that this is more likely to occur with agents that have greater lipophilicity, which enables easier penetration of the central nervous system. To my knowledge, differential susceptibility to depression with various β-blockers has not been demonstrated. Because depression is a subjective symptom that often waxes and wanes in its manifestations, it is often difficult to assess the effect of antihypertensive therapy. With the availability of newer antidepressant drugs such as the serotonin uptake inhibitors, which appear to have less effect on blood pressure than the tricyclic agents, it may be more effective to treat depressive symptoms medically than to mount repeated trials of antihypertensive agents and their subsequent withdrawal.

References

1.   Modan M, Almog S, Fuchs Z, et al: Obesity, glucose intolerance, hyperinsulinemia, and response to antihypertensive drugs. *Hypertension* 1991;17:565-573.

2.   Goode GK, Miller JP, Heagerty AM: Hyperlipidemia, hypertension, and coronary heart disease. *Lancet* 1995;345:362-365.

3.   Reaven GM: Role of insulin resistance in human disease. *Diabetes* 1988;37:1595-1607.

4.   Savage DD, Garrison RJ, Kannel WB, et al: The spectrum of left ventricular hypertrophy in a general population sample: the Framingham study. *Circulation* 1987;75:26-33.

5.   Ferrannini E, Buzzigoli G, Bonadonna R, et al: Insulin resistance in essential hypertension. *N Engl J Med* 1987;317:350-357.

6.   Baron AD, Laakso M, Brechtel G, et al: Mechanism of insulin resistance in insulin-dependent diabetes mellitus: a major role for reduced skeletal muscle blood flow. *J Clin Endocrinol Metab* 1991;73:637-643.

7.   Rochini AP, Key J, Bondie D, et al: The effect of weight loss on the sensitivity of blood pressure to sodium in obese adolescents. *N Engl J Med* 1989;321:580-585.

8.   National High Blood Pressure Education Program Working Group: report on hypertension in diabetes. *Hypertension* 1994; 23:145-158.

9.   Dominguez LJ, Weinberger MH, Cefalu WT, et al: Doxazosin improves insulin sensitivity and lowers blood pressure in type II diabetic hypertensives with no changes in tyrosine kinase activity or insulin binding. *Am J Hypertens* 1995;8:528-532.

10. Weinberger MH: Antihypertensive therapy and lipids: evidence, mechanisms and implications. *Arch Intern Med* 1985; 145:1102-1105.

11. Leary WP, Reyes AJ, Acosta-Barrios TN, et al: Captopril once daily as monotherapy in patients with hyperuricaemia and essential hypertension. *Lancet* 1985;1:1277-1279.

12. Nakashima M, Uedmatsa T, Kosuge K, et al: Pilot study of the uricosuric effect of DuP 753, a new angiotensin II receptor antagonist, in healthy subjects. *Eur J Clin Pharmacol* 1992; 42:333-335.

13. Cerasola G, Cottone S, D'Ignoto G, et al: Micro-albuminuria as a predictor of cardiovascular damage in essential hypertension. *J Hypertens* 1989;7:332-333.

14. Bakris GL: Blood pressure control and progression of diabetic nephropathy: are all antihypertensive drugs created equal? *Kidney* 1994;3:61-62.

15. Dahlof B, Pennert K, Hansson L: Reversal of left ventricular hypertrophy in hypertensive patients: a meta-analysis of 109 treatment studies. *Am J Hypertens* 1992;5:95-110.

16. Furberg CD, Psaty BM, Meyer JV: Dose-related increase in mortality in patients with coronary artery disease. *Circulation* 1995;92:1326-1331.

17. Cohn JN, Johnson G, Ziesche S, et al: A comparison of enalapril with hydralazine-isosorbide dinitrate in the treatment of chronic congestive heart failure. *N Engl J Med* 1991;325:303-310.

18. Deedwania PC: Angiotensin-converting enzyme inhibitors in congestive heart failure. *Arch Intern Med* 1990;150:1798-1805.

19. Pfeffer MA, Braunwald E, Moy LA, et al: Effect of captopril on mortality in patients with left ventricular dysfunction after myocardial infarction: results of the Survival and Ventricular Enlargement Trial. *N Engl J Med* 1992;327:669-677.

20. Siscovick DS, Raghunathan TE, Psaty BM, et al: Diuretic therapy and the risk of primary cardiac arrest. *N Engl J Med* 1994;330:1852-1857.

21. Hoes AW, Grobbee DE, Lubsen J, et al: Diuretics, β-blockers, and the risk for sudden cardiac death in hypertensive patients. *Ann Intern Med* 1995;123:481-487.

22. Fraunfelder FT, Barker AF: Respiratory effects of timolol. *N Engl J Med* 1984;311:1441-1444.

23. Henrich WL: Nephrotoxicity of nonsteroidal anti-inflammatory agents. In: Schrier RW, Gottschalk CW, eds. *Diseases of the Kidney.* Boston, Little Brown, 1993, pp 1203-1218.

Chapter 10

Complicated Hypertension

Treatment-Resistant Hypertension

Occasionally, blood pressure remains elevated despite what appears to be an adequate antihypertensive drug regimen. Evaluation of treatment-resistant blood pressure presents a distinct challenge to the clinician because the causes may be varied. They include noncompliance with prescribed regimens, improper choice of drugs, pharmacologic interference of other agents, secondary hypertension, true refractoriness, or a rare case of ineffective drug therapy. Identifying the cause of treatment resistance is often difficult because evaluating these factors can be confrontational, particularly with noncompliance and interfering agents.

The most common cause of treatment resistance is failure to adhere to the prescribed regimen. Some patients simply will not take medication as requested or may take it in reduced amount or frequency. This is the most difficult problem to identify because few patients admit to such behavior. Examination of dates on prescription vials or communication with the pharmacist may provide information about the timeliness of refilling medications. Table 10-1 outlines strategies to increase patient compliance.

For some patients, the perceived increase in urinary frequency from sporadic use of diuretics or from short-acting agents taken once or twice daily often leads to noncompliance with the therapeutic regimen. Reassuring the patient,

Table 10-1: Tips to Reduce Noncompliance

- make patient aware of the potential risks of uncontrolled hypertension
- explain the variety of therapeutic options available
- identify resources available to help achieve lifestyle modification
- inform patient that side effects may occur with any treatment
- encourage patient to report side effects or problems with medication
- offer remedies for side effects or suggest other therapy
- consider the financial implications of therapy
- use long-acting drugs
- incorporate pill taking with routine daily activities

explaining the need to include diuretics as a part of the therapeutic regimen, and using long-acting agents that do not promote continued marked diuresis after the initial days of treatment may all help to minimize noncompliance. A clinician should suspect noncompliance when agents often associated with certain physiologic effects are prescribed in therapeutically effective doses and those effects are not observed, such as if the pulse rate fails to decline with appropriately prescribed doses of β-adrenergic blocking drugs. However, the effectiveness of drugs can be influenced by other factors. Cigarette smoking, alcohol consumption, or hyperthyroidism often increase heart rate in the presence of β-blockers. The ingestion of medication with food having high fiber content or in the presence of gastrointestinal disease may also influence absorption of drugs.

As mentioned in the chapters on drug therapy, pseudotolerance to antihypertensive therapy may result from extracellular fluid volume expansion secondary to salt and water retention induced by vasodilators and other nondiuretic antihypertensive drugs. This can be remedied by the administration of effective diuretics. Another cause of apparent treatment resistance is the use of multiple drugs with similar mechanisms of action. For example, using central agonists and peripheral sympathetic antagonists in combination with a β-adrenergic blocker may be less effective than adding a drug of the vasodilator group and a small dose of diuretic. Similarly, the use of several vasodilators in combination, such as hydralazine, peripheral α_1-blockers, and calcium channel entry blockers without a diuretic or antisympathetic or β-blocking drug, may not be effective.

Pharmacologic interference can result in blood pressure apparently refractory to antihypertensive therapy when agents such as nonsteroidal anti-imflammatory drugs (NSAIDs) are used, which promote sodium and water retention. These drugs can also blunt the effectiveness of several antihypertensive agents such as diuretics, angiotensin-converting enzyme (ACE) inhibitors, and β-blockers. Moreover, these agents are often available over-the-counter, and the physician may not be aware of their use. Because they are given for a variety of problems, corticosteroids can also interfere with the effectiveness of antihypertensive regimens, as can other drugs such as thyroid replacement therapy, estrogens and oral contraceptives, cyclosporine, some antidepressants, and sympathomimetic agents (eg, diet aids, decongestants).

Secondary forms of hypertension may also be treatment resistant. When a reasonable therapeutic regimen fails to significantly lower blood pressure, evaluation for a secondary form of hypertension may be appropriate (see Chapter 4).

Malignant Hypertension

Secondary forms of hypertension are often severe and present as accelerated or malignant hypertension. This phase of blood pressure elevation, which can occur with primary or secondary forms of hypertension, denotes extensive and life-threatening vascular involvement. The distinction between accelerated and malignant designations is based on the severity of the vascular manifestations and not the level of blood pressure. No specific numeric criteria exist for the diagnosis of malignant hypertension because it may occur with blood pressure as low as 160/100 mm Hg and yet be absent with levels of 250/150 mm Hg. The diagnosis of malignant hypertension rests on elevation of blood pressure *and* evidence of end-organ failure involving the brain, heart, or kidneys. Thus, evidence of encephalopathy (ranging from headaches to coma), acute pulmonary edema, congestive heart failure, or renal failure in a patient with hypertension calls for immediate intervention. Unfortunately, discriminating between stroke and hypertensive encephalopathy is often difficult, and usually requires retrospective assessment after improvement of the cerebral symptoms after a period of blood pressure reduction. Papilledema is typical in hypertensive encephalopathy, but is not always discernible.[1]

Although malignant hypertension requires immediate evaluation and treatment, it does not require precipitous and uncontrolled blood pressure reduction.[2-4] A physical evaluation, laboratory tests, and electrocardiographic studies should be performed and historic information should be obtained to shed light on a possible etiology and on any issues about treatment. The laboratory studies should focus on renal function, electrolytes, and complete blood count. Then, the blood pressure should be lowered gradually using constant monitoring techniques to prevent compromise of end-organ function by precipitous lowering of pressure.[2-4] The rate and degree of blood pressure reduction depend on the initial level, evidence of end-organ dysfunction, and other factors based on history, laboratory evaluation, and physical examination. Usually, it will be necessary to admit the patient to an intensive care unit where blood pressure, pulse, and cardiovascular status can be constantly monitored. A variety of agents can be used to gradually reduce blood pressure.

Careful control typically requires the use of parenteral agents. Sodium nitroprusside (Nipride) has long been used for this purpose.[5] It is administered by continuous intravenous drip, and requires constant blood pressure monitoring so that the rate of the infusion can be adjusted to maintain blood pressure in the desired range. It is prudent to reduce the blood pressure in gradual stages and then to observe the effect on end-organ function over several hours before attempting to return blood pressure to the normal range. A precipitous reduction in pressure could compromise autoregulation of cerebral or cardiac blood flow.

Because nitroprusside is a potent vasodilator, expansion of extracellular fluid volume and increased sympathetic nervous system activity invariably occur. Thus, effective diuretics, including parenteral agents, are usually necessary. In addition, if there are no contraindications such as congestive heart failure, β-adrenergic blockers may be needed to decrease the elevation of heart rate secondary to sympathetic stimulation with nitroprusside. Intravenous β-blockers such as esmolol (Brevibloc®), which has a short half-life, can be titrated to a specific heart rate target. A variety of other agents can be administered parenterally for rapid blood pressure reduction. Potent, short-acting agents such as immediate-release nifedipine should not be used because of the potential for uncontrolled hypotension and resultant catastrophic vascular compromise, myocardial infarction, stroke, and death.[3]

When marked elevations of blood pressure occur without evidence of end-organ failure, there is less urgency for blood pressure reduction. The patient has probably had marked elevated pressure for some time and, thus, it is reasonable to reduce blood pressure over 1 to 2 hours during observation and evaluation. This approach does not require an intensive care unit for parenteral drug administration and monitoring. Such individuals can be evaluated and then given oral antihypertensive medications while being observed in the office, clinic, or outpatient setting. Determining which drugs are likely to have the greatest efficacy and benefit depends on several factors, including demographic characteristics such as age and race. The presence of certain disorders (see Chapter 9) may provide information about which agents may be preferable or best avoided. Most oral agents have an onset of action of 30 to 60 minutes (except for the clonidine skin patch, which requires 18 to 24 hours). Therefore, it is not necessary to initiate treatment with short-acting drugs. The full effect may take repeated doses and combination therapy to control blood pressure at the desired levels. However, it is usually possible to initiate therapy with a single agent in the outpatient setting and have the patient return at an appropriate time for follow-up, dose titration, or addition of other drugs. In general, it is preferable to initiate treatment with an intermediate or long-acting calcium channel entry blocker or ACE inhibitor because of their efficacy and safety. Short-acting calcium channel entry blockers should *not* be used. In the case of ACE inhibitors or angiotensin II receptor blockers (ARBs), diuretics are often required to enhance the antihypertensive response in older subjects or in African Americans.[6]

Several approaches that deserve comment have become popular for the treatment of accelerated or malignant hypertension. The use of immediate-release nifedipine was already mentioned and should never be used for this indication because of the dangers associated with it.[3] Another technique is the administration of oral clonidine (Catapres®) in an initial dose of 0.1 or 0.2 mg and then repeated every hour (usually in additional doses of 0.1 mg) until blood pressure declines to the desired level. A recent study indicated that the same blood pressure level was achieved after 6 hours with a single dose as was achieved with repeated dosing.[7] However, extreme somnolence and even an inability to be aroused are dose-dependent side effects of this agent. Thus, when the blood pressure is satisfactorily lowered, the patient may be unable to leave the medical care facility except with the assistance of others.

Clinicians should recognize that patients with accelerated or malignant hypertension are rarely unidentified new hypertensives. This phase of hypertension is invariably associated with inadequate treatment, frank noncompliance, a secondary form of hypertension, or drug interaction. Thus, an educational effort often helps in avoiding a recurrence in previously identified hypertensive patients.

Hypertension in Pregnancy

When hypertension occurs in a pregnant woman, the initial concern is whether the elevated blood pressure antedated pregnancy or represents pregnancy-related hypertension. Thus, hypertension that occurs during pregnancy often poses a diagnostic dilemma. Because pregnant women are often young, they may have few reasons to seek routine medical care before they become pregnant, and a blood pressure history is often not available. Hypertension *of* pregnancy does not typically occur before the 26th week of gestation. However, inaccurate prediction of gestational duration or failure to seek medical care early in pregnancy may make the onset of blood pressure elevation difficult to evaluate. Thus, it is often not until the blood pressure returns to normal in the postpartum period that a diagnosis of pregnancy-induced hypertension can be confidently made. In any event, blood pressure elevation during pregnancy is an important complication that requires special consideration.

Secondary forms of hypertension rarely occur in pregnancy. Two such forms have been associated with disastrous outcomes for the mother and fetus—Cushing's syndrome and pheochromocytoma.[8,9] In the former, menstrual dysfunction is common so that conception is difficult. Measurement of free cortisol in the urine is probably the most accurate way of identifying this condition, because plasma cortisol levels may be increased during pregnancy as the result of an increase in steroid-binding proteins. Pheochromocytoma is detected using the urinary tests mentioned in Chapter 4. Once the diagnosis of either of these forms of secondary hypertension is made, effective intervention is required to avoid maternal and fetal mortality. Pheochromocytoma is best treated surgically, whereas the treatment of Cushing's syndrome depends on the etiology (see Chapter 4). Renal vascular hypertension may also occur during pregnancy.[10] This can be treated with antihypertensive agents and careful monitoring of both blood pressure and renal function until after delivery, when decisions can be made about definitive treatment of the renal vascular lesion. When primary aldosteronism occurs in pregnant women, the manifestations are often improved because of the antialdosterone effects of elevated levels of progesterone.[11] Thus, a decrease in blood pressure and blunting of the hypokalemic alkalosis often occur, which become worse after delivery. The diagnosis can be made as outlined in Chapter 4. Evaluation and treatment can often be deferred until after delivery.

A patient known to have hypertension who wishes to become pregnant should be informed of the increased risk to her health as well as to that of the fetus. Because the true teratogenic potential of antihypertensive agents is not well known, and because the most vulnerable period is early in the pregnancy, hypertensive patients should be asked to discontinue antihypertensive drugs and pursue nonpharmacologic therapy (see Chapter 5) before attempting to become pregnant. This is usually not as risky as it may sound in cases of mild to moderate hypertension. Blood pressure normally declines in the first trimester of pregnancy, when the greatest adverse effect on fetal development might be anticipated, and then rises during the second and third trimesters, when the risk of drug treatment may be less.

The management of a pregnant patient with hypertension requires more frequent evaluation than for a nonhypertensive patient. Because blood pressure can rise precipitously and the symptoms of eclampsia can develop rapidly, even at relatively modest elevations of blood pressure, home blood pressure monitoring is often useful, either by the patient or by another trained individual between scheduled follow-up visits. Renal function and the presence of proteinuria should also be carefully monitored.

When drug treatment of hypertension is required during pregnancy, choosing the appropriate agent is often more difficult.[12] There are few adequate carefully controlled studies of antihypertensive agents used during pregnancy. It is clear that ACE inhibitors and ARBs should not be used or should be discontinued immediately in the event of pregnancy because of the adverse experience with ACE inhibitors during pregnancy. There is no relevant information about the use of angiotensin II receptor antagonists; however, because of the adverse effects of ACE inhibitors, ARBs should not be used in pregnant women. Diuretic treatment is also not advisable unless mandated by renal failure and obvious fluid retention. Pedal edema during the second and third trimesters of pregnancy is more often related to venous compression by the enlarging uterus than to true fluid retention.

Because the chief pathophysiologic abnormality in pregnant women with hypertension is vasoconstriction and increased vascular resistance, the use of drugs directed against this component is usually effective in lowering blood pressure.[12] Hydralazine (Apresoline®) was used in the past for this purpose. However, the short duration of action of this agent, which requires t.i.d. to q.i.d. dosing, and its adverse effects (headache, nausea, vomiting, tachycardia) have lessened its use. Peripheral α_1-adrenergic receptor blockers such as prazosin (Minipress®), terazosin (Hytrin®), and doxazosin (Cardura®) are preferred. Prazosin must be given t.i.d., but the other two are effective once a day. Beta-adrenergic receptor blockers can also be used, but caution is required when the patient is near term because these agents can interfere with labor or cause fetal bradycardia. The centrally acting α-agonists are also used, but the resulting lethargy and dry mouth have been bothersome to many patients.

Another agent with a long history in the treatment of hypertension during pregnancy is α-methyldopa. Its major limitations are drowsiness, the potential to cause hepatic dysfunction, and the necessity of t.i.d. dosage. There is little information about the effects of calcium channel entry blockers in pregnancy. Intuitively, it would seem best to avoid those that could induce fetal bradycardia.

Hypertension and Renal Disease

Renal dysfunction is common among patients with hypertension.[13] It is often difficult to ascertain whether the blood pressure elevation preceded or resulted from the renal disease when the patient is first seen and abnormalities of both are present. As previously discussed, a variety of renal abnormalities can lead to elevated blood pressure. The mechanism for this may be either extracellular fluid volume expansion that results from impaired renal excretory function, or increased production of vasoconstrictor substances such as renin and angiotensin II, and occasionally, a combination of these factors. The former is best treated with diuretics, recognizing that thiazide diuretics are less effective when renal impairment is present and that loop agents must usually be used. ACE inhibitors and angiotensin II receptor antagonists would seem to be appropriate therapeutic options for the renin-angiotensin-mediated vasoconstriction. However, when renal perfusion is reduced, glomerular filtration depends on renin-angiotensin II-induced efferent arteriolar constriction. Thus, the use of agents that interfere with this action may worsen renal function.[13]

Hypertension is common in diabetic renal disease, and blood pressure control is necessary to prevent or control its progression. Proteinuria is often a harbinger of diabetic renal disease. Evidence suggests that strict blood pressure control, particularly with ACE inhibitors, can delay the onset or slow the progression of diabetic nephropathy.[13] Recent observations indicate that the reduction of blood pressure to levels below 140/90 may be beneficial in preventing the development or progression of diabetic renal disease. Studies are in progress to determine whether ARBs have a similar effect. Proteinuria also appears to predict renal and other vascular events in hypertensive patients without diabetes. There is no information about the differential benefits of specific antihypertensive agents on either the renal disease or the vascular sequelae.

Hypertension in Children and Adolescents

When blood pressure elevation occurs in childhood, it is often associated with an identifiable cause, as primary (essential) hypertension is uncommon in children. The most likely causes involve the kidneys (eg, renal parenchymal disease, renal vascular disease, renal trauma, renal tumors), the adrenal glands (eg, pheochromocytoma, primary aldosteronism), and coarctation of the aorta. Iatrogenic causes from corticosteroid treatment or excessive doses of thyroid hormone can also be a factor. Most of these secondary forms can be treated. Occasionally, the abuse of licorice, corticosteroids, amphetamines, cocaine, or other agents may cause elevated blood pressure in this group. Although less common in children than in adults, primary (essential) hypertension may also occur. For a variety of reasons, nonpharmacologic therapy should be the initial approach. Because many such children are obese, an exercise and weight loss program may be sufficient.[14] Other dietary recommendations, outlined in Chapter 5, are also appropriate. When drug therapy is required, the physician must consider the potential effects of the drugs chosen. Many agents influence central nervous system or hormonal balance, and consultation with a specialist in pediatrics or pediatric pharmacology may be necessary to avoid unwanted side effects or growth and development.

Hypertension in the Elderly

The prevalence of hypertension increases with age.[15] Elevated blood pressure is one of the most common long-term disorders in older patients and one of the major modifiable risk factors for cardiovascular disease in this group. Moreover, there are special therapeutic considerations in elderly patients with hypertension based on pathophysiologic, behavioral, economic, and cultural differences with their younger cohorts. A loss of elasticity of vascular tissues occurs with age, which contributes to the increased vascular resistance and decreased cardiac contractility typically found in older hypertensives. Structural and functional changes in renal capacity, alterations in hepatic metabolism, and changes in sympathetic nervous system activity or response further influence the development of hypertension, the effects and metabolism of drugs, and the ability to compensate for hemodynamic changes in the elderly.

Beause older patients have fewer defenses against excessive volume depletion, azotemia, dehydration, and orthostatic hypotension are more likely to occur with diuretic therapy. In addition, hyponatremic responses to such drugs are more common in the elderly. Hypokalemia with diuretic therapy is common, perhaps abetted by a diet that is reduced in potassium-rich foods (fresh fruits and vegetables). Left ventricular enlargement and coronary artery disease may predispose older patients to the risk of arrhythmias, which can be compounded by hypokalemia. Constipation is another common problem that can be aggravated by many antihypertensive drugs, particularly the calcium channel entry blockers and diuretics.

Many older patients have metabolic problems such as gout, diabetes, and lipid disorders that can be affected by the choice of antihypertensive drug therapy. In general, diuretics and β-blockers have an adverse effect on these conditions; peripheral α_1-adrenergic receptor blockers are beneficial; and the other blood pressure-lowering agents are neutral. In hypertensive patients who also have angina or congestive heart failure, special consideration must be given to the choice of drugs, as discussed in Chapter 9.

Depression and memory problems are common in older patients, so agents with central nervous system effects should be avoided. Simplification of the drug regimen is very important because multiple drugs and multiple doses portend disaster or noncompliance for any patient, particularly the elderly. Drugs taken once a day at breakfast or when brushing teeth are most likely to be effective.

Polypharmacy may be yet another confounding element in the treatment of some elderly hypertensives. Older patients often have upper respiratory or musculoskeletal and joint disorders for which they take a variety of prescription or over-the-counter medications, with the potential for interaction with antihypertensive agents or for adverse effects on renal function.

Older men often have benign prostatic hyperplasia. A history of urinary difficulty that includes hesitancy, dysuria, dribbling, and particularly nocturia are common manifestations of obstructive uropathy. In hypertensive patients, these symptoms are sometimes blamed on the antihypertensive medications, and noncompliance results. Such symptoms require evaluation by digital rectal examination, measurement of prostate-specific antigen (PSA) and, if indicated, prostatic ultrasound, biopsy, and even surgical intervention. In patients for whom surgery is not deemed urgent, a trial of medical management for symptomatic relief is often chosen.

Table 10-2: Combination Drugs for Hypertension

Diuretic Combinations

amiloride (5 mg) + HCTZ (50 mg)

spironolactone (25, 50 mg) + HCTZ (25, 50 mg)
(Aldactazide®)

triamterene (37.5, 50, 75 mg) + HCTZ (25, 50 mg)
(Dyazide®, Maxzide®)

ACE Inhibitors + Calcium Channel Antagonists

benazepril (10, 20 mg) + amlodipine (2.5, 5 mg) (Lotrel®)

enalapril (5 mg) + diltiazem (180 mg) (Teczem®)

enalapril (5 mg) + felodipine (5 mg) (Lexxel®)

trandolapril (1, 2, 4 mg) + verapamil (180, 240) (Tarka®)

Angiotensin Receptor Antagonists + Diuretic

irbesartan (150 mg) + HCTZ (12.5 mg) (Avalide®)

losartan (50 mg) + HCTZ (12.5 mg) (Hyzaar®)

valsartan (80, 160 mg) + HCTZ (12.5 mg) (Diovan HCT®)

Beta-Adrenergic Blockers + Diuretics

atenolol (50, 100 mg) + chlorthalidone (25 mg)
(Tenoretic®)

bisoprolol (2.5, 5, 10 mg) + HCTZ (6.25 mg) (Ziac®)

metoprolol (50, 100 mg) + HCTZ (25, 50 mg)
(Lopressor HCT®)

nadolol (40, 80 mg) + bendroflumethazide (5 mg)
(Corzide®)

propranolol (40, 80 mg) + HCTZ (25 mg) (Inderide®)

timolol (10 mg) + HCTZ (25 mg) (Timolide®)

Finasteride (Proscar®) can reduce an enlarged prostate. Results with this agent generally require several months of treatment. A particularly useful alternative for hypertensive patients is the administration of α_1-adrenergic receptor blockers such as prazosin (Minipress®), terazosin (Hytrin®), or doxazosin (Cardura®).[16] The latter two agents are

Other Combinations

clonidine (0.1, 0.2, 0.3 mg) + chlorthalidone (15 mg) (Combipres®)

guanethidine (10 mg) + HCTZ (25 mg) (Esimil®)

hydralazine (25, 50, 100 mg) + HCTZ (25, 50 mg) (Apresazide®)

methyldopa (250, 500 mg) + HCTZ (15, 25, 30, 50 mg) (Aldoril®)

prazosin (1, 2, 5 mg) + PTZ (0.5 mg) (Minizide®)

reserpine (0.125, 0.25 mg) + HCTZ (25, 50 mg) (Hydropres®)

reserpine (0.125, 0.25 mg) + CT (25, 50 mg) (Demi-Regrofon®)

reserpine (0.125, 0.25 mg) + CTZ (250, 500 mg) (Diupres®)

reserpine (0.1 mg) + hydralazine (25 mg) + HCTZ (15 mg) (Ser-Ap-Es®)

HCTZ = hydrochlorothiazide
CT = chlorthalidone
CTZ = chlorothiazide
PTZ = polythiazide

generally effective when given once a day, whereas prazosin requires multiple dosing because of its short duration of action. These agents work by decreasing sympathetic tone at the level of the bladder sphincter rather than by directly reducing prostate size. The major limitations of α_1-blocker treatment are the risks of orthostatic hypotension and dizziness, which increase in the elderly. These risks can be minimized in several ways. Initiation of therapy should begin with the lowest dose, preferably with the first dose given at bedtime along with a warning about the risk of suddenly changing position. Some physicians prefer that patients continue to take their dose at bedtime, not just the first dose. Orthostatic dizziness may also occur more often in patients who receive diuretic therapy.

The upward titration of the dose should be slow, maintaining a given dose for 7 to 14 days before increasing it. The increase should be based on both the blood pressure response and the response of the symptoms of obstructive uropathy. If blood pressure declines excessively while the α_1-blocker is being titrated, it may be possible to reduce the dose of other medications being taken for blood pressure. The major improvements in urinary symptoms with α_1-blockers are a reduction in urinary hesitancy, improved force of the urinary stream, and a notable decrease in the frequency of nocturia.

Isolated Systolic Hypertension

Systolic pressure that is persistently above 140 mm Hg and diastolic that is below 90 mm Hg is described as isolated systolic hypertension. Because this usually occurs in older patients, its cause is assumed to be the result of sclerotic blood vessels and the increased resistance associated with aging. It can also occur in hyperthyroidism and other high output states. In the past, because of the common association between isolated systolic hypertension and age, it was erroneously assumed that the higher systolic pressure was necessary to provide adequate tissue perfusion. Epidemiologic evidence convincingly demonstrated that the level of systolic pressure, irrespective of diastolic, is the best predictor of virtually every form of cardiovascular event, including stroke, myocardial infarction, left ventricular hypertrophy, congestive heart failure, and renal failure.[17] Studies have recently been conducted in this population to examine the benefit of reducing isolated increase in systolic pressure. The results indicate that a decrease in cardiovascular events is an overwhelming benefit when systolic pressure is lowered.[18] Physicians can now recommend lowering systolic pressure to at least 160 mm Hg when it is initially 180 mm Hg or higher, and targeting reduction to the 140 mm Hg range when baseline values are 160 to 180 mm Hg. Typically, lowering systolic pressure in patients with isolated systolic hypertension does not usually lead to an excessive reduction in the already normal diastolic pressure.

A few trials have been conducted using diuretics and β-adrenergic blockers as primary treatment. The use of potassium-sparing diuretic combinations has been shown to be more beneficial than the use of diuretics alone. A recent trial with a dihydropyridine calcium channel blocker, nitrendipine, demonstrated a significant reduction in stroke in elderly patients.[19] Because of the special concerns in the elderly, it is important to use low doses of drugs and to monitor for potential adverse effects, particularly those to which the elderly are more susceptible. The use of combination therapy by adding small doses of different antihypertensive agents is likely to provide safe and effective blood pressure reduction in this group of patients as in other hypertensives.

Combination Drug Therapy

The most recent report of the Joint National Committee (JNC VI) has included combination drug therapy among the initial therapeutic options. The rationale for including combinations is based on the additive antihypertensive effect when agents of two different drug classes are used, as well as the improved efficacy at lower doses than would be required for monotherapy. Since side effects are often dose dependent, the ability to achieve blood pressure control with low-dose combinations may often reduce side effects when compared to monotherapy at higher doses. A combination may also improve compliance by reducing the number of pills required. Certain combinations can ameliorate side effects of one of the components. Examples are the decrease in pedal edema when benazepril is added to amlodipine (Lotrel®) or the blunting of hypokalemia and hyperuricemia when ACE inhibitors are combined with diuretics (Capozide®, Vaseretic®). Table 10-2 lists the combination agents available in the United States at the time of this writing.

References

1. McGregor E, Isles CG, Jay JL, et al: Retinal changes in malignant hypertension. *Br Med J* 1986;292:233-234.

2. Ledingham JG, Rajagopalan B: Cerebral complications in the treatment of accelerated hypertension. *Q J Med* 1979;48:25-41.

3. Noble-Orazio E, Sterzl R: Cerebral ischemia after nifedipine treatment. *Br Med J* 1981;283:948-950.

4. Haas DC, Streeten DH, Kim RC, et al: Death from cerebral hypoperfusion during nitroprusside treatment of acute angiotensin-dependent hypertension. *Am J Med* 1983;75:1071-1076.

5. Page IH, Corcoran AC, Dustan HP, et al: Cardiovascular actions of sodium nitroprusside in animal and hypertensive patients. *Circulation* 1955;11:188-198.

6. Weinberger MH: Blood pressure and metabolic responses to hydrochlorothiazide, captopril and the combination in black and white mild-to-moderate hypertensive patients. *J Cardiovasc Pharm* 1985;7:S52-S55.

7. Zeller KR, Kuhnert LV, Matthews C: Rapid reduction of severe asymptomatic hypertension. *Arch Intern Med* 1989;149:2186-2189.

8. Aron DC, Schnall AM, Sheeler LR: Cushing's syndrome and pregnancy. *Am J Obstet Gynecol* 1990;162:244-252.

9. Lamming GD, Symonds EM, Rubin PC: Pheochromocytoma in pregnancy: still a cause of maternal death. *Clin Exp Hyper* 1990;B9:57-68.

10. Easterling TR, Brateng D, Goldman ML, et al: Renal vascular hypertension during pregnancy. *Obstet Gynecol* 1991;78:921-925.

11. Ehrlich EN, Laves M, Lugibihl K, et al: Progesterone-aldosterone interrelationships in pregnancy. *J Lab Clin Med* 1962; 59:588-593.

12. Barron WM, Lindheimer MD: Management of hypertension during pregnancy. In: Laragh JH, Brenner BM, eds. *Hypertension: Pathophysiology, Diagnosis, and Management*, 2nd ed. New York, Raven Press, 1995, pp 2427-2450.

13. Preston RA, Singer I, Epstein M: Renal parenchymal hypertension: current concepts of pathogenesis and management. *Arch Intern Med* 1996;156:602-611.

14. Rocchini AP, Key J, Bondie D, et al: The effect of weight loss on the sensitivity of blood pressure to sodium in obese adolescents. *N Engl J Med* 1989;321:580-585.

15. The Joint National Committee on Prevention, Detection, Evaluation and Treatment of High Blood Pressure: The sixth report (JNC VI). *Arch Intern Med* 1997;157:2413-2446.

16. Ramsay JW, Scott GI, Whitfield HN: A double-blind controlled trial of a new $\alpha\text{-}_1$ blocking drug in the treatment of bladder outflow obstruction. *Br J Urol* 1985;57:657-659.

17. Kannel WB, Castelli WP, McNamara PM, et al: Role of blood pressure in the development of congestive heart failure. The Framingham study. *N Engl J Med* 1972;287:781-787.

18. Systolic Hypertension in the Elderly Research Group: implications of the systolic hypertension in the elderly program. *Hypertension* 1993;21:335-343.

19. Staessen JA, Fagard R, Thijs L, et al, for the Systolic Hypertension-Europe (Syst-Eur) Trial Investigators: Morbidity and mortality in the placebo-controlled European trial on isolated systolic hypertension in the elderly. *Lancet* 1997;360:757-764.

Index

A

Midamor® 74, 78

Minipress® 36, 56, 84, 86, 106, 114, 128, 132

Minizide® 133

minoxidil (Loniten®) 84, 86, 110, 111

Moduretic® 53, 74, 78

moexipril (Univasc™) 86

monoamine oxidase (MAO) inhibitors 103

Monopril® 86

monotherapy 107, 135

"moon" facies 42

multiple endocrine neoplasia (MEN) syndrome 41, 54

murmurs 37

muscle weakness 41

Mykrox® 75

myocardial infarction 9, 11, 12, 53, 83, 89, 92, 94, 101, 105, 108, 110, 111, 123, 134

myocardial ischemia 10, 83, 92, 112

N

nadolol (Corgard®) 99

nadolol + bendroflumethazide (Corzide®) 132

nasal congestion 99

nasal sprays 33

nasal stuffiness 93, 100

National Heart, Lung, and Blood Institute 14

natriuresis 80, 93

nausea 36, 77, 127

necrosis 55

nephrectomy 47, 59

neurofibromas 41, 42, 54

nicardipine (Cardene®) 88

nifedipine (Adalat® CC, Procardia XL®) 53, 88, 92, 94, 123, 124

Nipride 82, 123

nisoldipine (Sular®) 88

nitrendipine 92, 135

nitric oxide 19, 22, 25, 26, 28, 82, 105

nitroprusside (Nipride®) 26, 82, 83, 123

nocturia 36, 41, 85, 114, 131, 134

noncompliance 119, 120, 125, 131

nonsteroidal anti-inflammatory drugs (NSAIDs) 33, 79, 114, 121

norepinephrine 19, 22, 23, 26, 29, 55, 74, 103

NOTES

NOTES

NOTES